Procedures for Primary Care Practitioners

Procedures for Primary Care Practitioners

MARILYN WINTERTON EDMUNDS, RN, PhD, CRNP
Adult and Geriatric Nurse Practitioner
Associate Professor
Formerly Graduate Nurse Practitioner Program
University of Maryland
Baltimore, Maryland

MAREN STEWART MAYHEW, RN, MS, CRNP
Adult and Geriatric Nurse Practitioner
Assistant Professor
Formerly Graduate Nurse Practitioner Program
University of Maryland
Baltimore, Maryland

Foreword by
DAVID G. RORISON, MD, MBA
Chairman, Emergency Department
Mercy Medical Center
Baltimore, Maryland

Additional contributions by:
CARL ANDERSON, PAC
Clinical Coordinator/Instructor
Department of Physician Assistant Education
St. Louis University Medical Center
St. Louis, Missouri

Mosby

St. Louis Baltimore Boston Carlsbad Chicago Naples New York Philadelphia Portland
London Madrid Mexico City Singapore Sydney Tokyo Toronto Wiesbaden

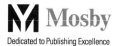

Mosby
Dedicated to Publishing Excellence

A Times Mirror
Company

Publisher: Nancy Coon
Editor: Robin Carter
Developmental Editor: Jeanne Allison
Project Manager: Linda McKinley
Editing and Production: Graphic World Publishing Services
Designer: Elizabeth Fett

A NOTE TO THE READER:

The author and publisher have made every attempt to check dosages and nursing content for accuracy. Because the science of pharmacology is continually advancing, our knowledge base continues to expand. Therefore we recommend that the reader always check product information for changes in dosage or administration before administering any medication. This is particularly important with new or rarely used drugs.

Printed in the United States of America

Composition by Graphic World, Inc.
Printing/binding by Rand McNally

Mosby–Year Book, Inc.
11830 Westline Industrial Drive
St. Louis, Missouri 63146

Library of Congress Cataloging-in-Publication Data

Procedures for the primary care practitioner/[edited by] Marilyn Winterton
   Edmunds, Maren Stewart Mayhew; foreword by David G. Rorison;
   additional contributions by Carl Anderson.—1st ed.
      p.   cm.
   Includes bibliographical references and index.
   ISBN 0-8151-3034-1
   1. Nurse practitioners—Handbooks, manuals, etc.   2. Primary care
(Medicine)—Handbooks, manuals, etc.   3. Ambulatory medical care—
Handbooks, manuals, etc.   I. Edmunds, Marilyn W.   II. Mayhew,
Maren Stewart.
   [DNLM: 1. Primary Nursing Care—methods.   2. Ambulatory Care—
methods—nurses' instruction.   3. Nurse Practitioners.   WY 101
P963 1996]
RT82.8.P76   1996
610.73—dc20
DNLM/DLC
for Library of Congress   95-40072
                                                                                      CIP

97   98   99   00   /   9   8   7   6   5   4   3   2

Contributors

Christy L. Crowther MS, CRNP
Adult Nurse Practitioner
Infectious Disease and Orthopedics
Private Practice
Severna Park, Maryland

Cindy Grandjean MS, CRNP
Adult Nurse Practitioner
Private Practice
College Park, Maryland

Laurie E. Scudder MS, CRNP
Pediatric Nurse Practitioner
Assistant Professor
USUHS Uniformed Services University of Health Sciences
Bethesda, Maryland

Diane Seibert MS, CRNP
Adult and OB/GYN Nurse Practitioner
Private Practice
Columbia, Maryland

Consultants

Pat Balassone MS, ANP
Ohio State University
Columbus, Ohio

Pam Cacchione MS, GNP
Washington University
St. Louis, Missouri

Marjorie Maddox ARNP
Adult Day Center
Louisville, Kentucky

Lana Riddle PhD, NP
Brigham Young University
Provo, Utah

Acknowledgments

We gratefully acknowledge the contributions of our patients, who were really our *teachers,* and whose final examinations we ultimately had to pass as we worked in the "real world."

We would like to extend a special thank you to Bill Mayhew for all of his help.

We also want to acknowledge the contributions of our former students who completed the research and wrote initial versions of these procedures. Their questions and ideas provided us with the stimulus to revise and compile those procedures commonly performed by primary care nurse practitioners and physicians assistants and to standardize the educational preparation of graduates in these areas.

Baker, Deborah L. RN, MS, CRNP
Benson, Happy L. MS, CRNP
Beyer, Anne M. MS, CRNP
Bishop, Barbara S. MS, CRNP, CNRN
Bishop, Mary M. MS, CPNP
Blaemire, Evelyn Booth. MS, CRNP
Bounds, Marybeth G. RN, MS, CPNP
Brazier, Alice M. MS, CRNP
Bronson, Kathie C. MS, CRNP
Childs, Susan E. MS, CRNP
Coffey, Timothy A. RN-CS, ANP
Cotton, Sandra L. MS, CRNP
Custer, Judy A. RN, MS, CRNP, NP-C
Denicoff, Andrea M. RN, MSN
Devine, Jane Marie. RN, MS, CPNP
Drake, D. Kim. MS, CRNP
Dunko, Laura Moy. MS, CRNP
Flanary, Robin Neale. MS, CRNP

Fong, Diane Orth. MS, CRNP
Forrest, Deborah C. MS, CRNP
Fox, Karen L. MS, ANP
Freeman, Patricia Y. MS, CRNP
Gallo, Lauren Ann. MS, CRNP
Gering, Joyce N. MS, CRNP
Goleta, Flordeliza D. MS, CRNP
Graef, Bobbi H. MS, OB-GYN/Adult CRNP
Grandjean, Cynthia K. MS, CRNP
Green, Debra J. MS, CRNP
Green, Kimberly A. MS, CRNP, CCRN
Gregory, Irma L. MS, CRNP, NNP
Harrison, Debra T. MS, CPNP
Herriott, Kathleen. MS, NP
Hooper, Sarah Lynne. MS, CRNP
Hoover, Angelita A. MS, CRNP
Horne, Theresa A. MS, CRNP

Hwu, Kathleen M. MS, CRNP
Kalendek, Michelle E. MS, CRNP
Keiler, Laura C. MS, CRNP
Koehler, Margaret Lynn. MS, CRNP
Kohl, Bonnie M. MS, CRNP
Korger, Elizabeth. MS, ANP-C
Lansinger, Beth Ann. MS, CRNP
Lemieux, M. Lauren. MS, CRNP
Locke, Solveig K. MS, CRNP
Maier, Beth L. MS, CRNP
Martin, Paul K. MHS, RN
Matthews, Douglas Craig. MS, CRNP
McLaughlin, Randie R. MS, CRNP
McLean, Gail B. MS, CRNP
McMurtry, Brenda Novella. MS, CANP
Millard, Shirley M. MS, CRNP
Minor, Karen L. MS, CRNP
Mutch, Amy E. MS, CRNP
Nalewaik, Kathleen Q. MS, CRNP
O'Donnell, Patricia B. MS, CRNP
Plum, Georgia L. MS, CRNP

Pries, Justine. MSN, CRNP
Quinn, Catherine. MS, CRNP
Rackson, Mary A. MS, CRNP
Sample, Shirley Jane. MS, CRNP
Scharnhorst, Susanne W. MS, CRNP
Seibert, Diane C. MS, CRNP
Shagena, Kathleen M. MS, CRNP
Shay, Laura E. MS, CANP
Skowronek, Mary P. MS, CRNP
Smithson, Marcia Ann. RN, MS, CRNP
Speis, Karen E. MS, CRNP
Staat, Edwin P. MS, CRNP
Staubs, Rebecca Riddle. MS, CRNP
Thomas, Philsamma. MS, CRNP
Tirtanadi, Laurie Jane. MS CRNP
Van Horn, Emily A. MS, CRNP
Wemmer, Jan C. MS, CRNP
Wendel, V. Inez. MS, CRNP
Whiteford, Beth A. MS, CRNP
Yi, Susan S. MS, CRNP

Foreword

Healthcare delivery is changing at a revolutionary rate. In response to market pressures, new partnerships and new practice patterns have developed in rapid, dramatic, and pervasive ways. This redefinition has forced organizations and practitioners to develop innovative ways to be more effective and more efficient in the care they provide. How to offer improved service, at a lower cost, with demonstrable quality outcomes, has become the goal of all healthcare providers.

In many instances these demands have led to an increased focus in three key areas—*primary care,* the establishment of new *partnerships,* (partnerships between hospitals, hospitals and providers, and between varied providers), and the development of *new skill sets* for healthcare workers. The complex challenge of providing heightened value to patients and insurers, while maintaining an appropriate balance between quality and cost in this environment, has for obvious reasons placed midlevel practitioners in the spotlight. Now more than ever, physician practices, hospitals, and HMOs are depending on nurse practitioners and physician assistants as a quality driven solution to these market pressures. Value is defined by quality and cost. Those providers satisfying both these variables will be clearly part of the future healthcare equation and part of the solution. It is the ability of nurse practitioners and physician assistants to provide effective and more efficient primary health care that has made them pivotal and highly valued in many redesign and reform efforts.

This book is meant to serve as a reference and to further enhance the value of varied practitioners. It evolved from an analysis of current needs and future expectations. Currently, it is not unusual to be called on to perform simple office procedures in many primary care settings; in the future the demand is likely to be even greater. Those healthcare providers trained and accomplished in procedural skills, in addition to more traditional primary care, will further increase their contribution to any professional practice. In fact, in many practice settings it may be an absolute requirement for employment. Having practiced side-by-side with physician assistants and nurse practitioners for many years, I have long valued their diagnostic skills, patient advocacy, and ability to provide definitive care in many settings. The ability to support, or enhance, the procedural skillset is the goal of this collaborative text and should be the goal of the individual provider.

David G. Rorison, MD, MBA
Chairman, Emergency Department
Mercy Medical Center
Baltimore, Maryland

Preface

In the course of teaching nurse practitioners over the last 20 years, we have watched with interest the change in what primary care practitioners actually do when they assume clinical practice. Invariably, the reality of clinical practice is broader than what is taught in university programs. Academic curricula are often encumbered with bureaucracy and slow to change.

One specific area of content is difficult to teach in any formal program, and that concerns the office procedures found commonly in ambulatory care practices. There is wide diversity in the clinical sites employed for student education, and there is substantial difficulty in providing clinical experiences for the broad numbers of procedures. Many programs assume that graduates will learn procedures on the job and as dictated by the specific practice in which they work.

In an attempt to align curricular content more closely with practice, a few years ago we surveyed all the nurse practitioners within the state of Maryland to determine what procedures they were taught in their practitioner programs and which procedures they were actually utilizing in their clinical practices. We also asked questions about procedures which they were performing that were not commonly taught in nurse practitioner programs. Our conclusions as a result of this research were that there needed to be a stronger emphasis in graduate programs on a core of common procedures, but by far, graduates would continue to learn on the job the procedures required by their client population. What was needed was a reference text to outline the basic principles to which practitioners could refer. Thus, this text was born.

This book is designed for the advanced practitioner. It presumes that the clinician already has substantial experience and education. As such, this book, with few exceptions, does not cover basic nursing procedures and we refer practitioners back to basic nursing text for those types of procedures.

This is not a book designed for physicians. It is recognized that physicians' scope of practice often requires them to perform many acute care procedures in addition to the procedures listed here. There are a number of texts that clearly define the procedures performed by physicians. These texts usually do not cover the procedures performed by other practitioners.

This book is a reference text for nurse practitioners and physicians assistants who practice in primary care or emergency settings. Although state nurse practice acts may vary in what these types of practitioners are legally allowed to do, this text necessarily reflects the decisions of the editors about what practitioners are commonly allowed to do. It does not, therefore, include what we believe most primary care practitioners should not be doing.

The reader will note that there are some procedures which are noticeably absent. Specialized procedures that require specific training and certification, such as colposcopy, and Norplant insertion and removal, have been omitted. In addition, there are liability issues surrounding some procedures, including endometrial biopsy, which preclude including them in a book of common procedures. We encourage practitioners to attend the educational courses designed to give the didactic background and clinical supervision to prepare a practitioner in these procedures rather than to try to learn something out of a book.

Parts of this text may also be useful for certified nurse midwives and for physicians assistants. The physician assistant curriculum, in particular, commonly emphasizes more procedures than nursing programs. Whereas this text may provide a useful reference for physicians assistants who practice in primary care, emergency, or other ambulatory settings, there are other procedures that physician assistants may commonly perform, such as casting or placement of traction, that are not included.

Marilyn H. Edmunds
Maren Mayhew

Contents

Alphabetical Procedure List   xix

General Considerations for Every Procedure   xxi

Pediatric Considerations   xxv

Geriatric Considerations   xxvii

1 General Laboratory Procedures   1

2 Dermatologic Procedures   19

3 Eye, Ear, and Nose Procedures   99

4 Respiratory Procedures   137

5 Cardiovascular Procedures   153

6 Gastrointestinal Procedures   167

7 Musculoskeletal Procedures   199

8 Metabolic/Miscellaneous Procedures   221

9 Gynecologic Procedures   237

Appendices

A Checklist for Certification   273

B Bibliography   275

Detailed Contents

Alphabetical Procedure List *xix*

General Considerations for Every Procedure *xxi*

Pediatric Considerations *xxv*

Geriatric Considerations *xxvii*

1 General Laboratory Procedures *1*

Basic concepts of specimen collection *1*

Blood cultures *5*

Urinalysis *9*

Urine culture *13*

2 Dermatologic Procedures *19*

Skin lesion removal *19*

Anesthesia—local, topical, and digital nerve block *20*

Suturing simple lacerations *28*

Elliptical excision and biopsy *43*

Abscess incision and drainage *48*

Cyst removal *53*

Skin tag removal—cautery or snipping *56*

Wart removal—chemical and cryotherapy *59*

Ulcer debridement *68*

Wound care *71*

Fungal scraping—the KOH test *74*

Tick removal *79*

Corn and callus management *81*

Toenail care in the diabetic patient *84*

Ingrown toenail management   *88*
Subungual hematoma evacuation   *94*

3 Eye, Ear, and Nose Procedures   *99*

Removal of a foreign body from the eye   *99*
Treatment of corneal abrasion   *105*
Removal of a foreign body from the ear   *110*
Cerumen disimpaction   *113*
Ear piercing   *118*
Epistaxis and nasal packing   *122*
Removal of a foreign body from the nose   *130*

4 Respiratory Procedures   *137*

Nebulizer treatment   *137*
Spirometry   *139*
Oral airway insertion   *146*

5 Cardiovascular Procedures   *153*

Doppler ultrasound of lower extremities   *153*
Electrocardiogram   *158*
Continuous electrocardiography (Holter monitoring)   *163*

6 Gastrointestinal Procedures   *167*

Nasogastric tube insertion and removal   *167*
Gastric lavage   *174*
Anoscopy   *178*
Rectal prolapse reduction   *181*
Percutaneous endoscopic gastrostomy tube (PEG) management   *185*
Enteral tube feeding   *190*

7 Musculoskeletal Procedures   *199*

Fracture immobilization   *199*
Splinting—wrist and hand   *202*
Splinting—ankle sprains   *209*
Reduction of subluxed radial head   *218*

8 Metabolic/Miscellaneous Procedures   *221*

X-ray interpretation   *221*
Finger stick blood glucose   *224*
Bedside cystometrogram   *230*

9 Gynecologic Procedures *237*

Papanicolaou smear test *237*
The wet mount *242*
Treatment of condylomata acuminata *247*
Pessary use *253*
Diaphragm fitting *259*
Cervical cap placement *263*
Depo provera injection *268*

Appendices

A Checklist for Certification *273*
B Bibliography *275*

Index *277*

Alphabetical Procedure List

Abscess Incision and Drainage   *48*

Anesthesia—Local, Topical, and Digital Nerve Block   *20*

Anoscopy   *178*

Basic Concepts of Specimen Collection   *1*

Bedside Cystometrogram   *230*

Blood Cultures   *5*

Cerumen Disimpaction   *113*

Cervical Cap Placement   *263*

Continuous Electrocardiography (Holter Monitoring)   *163*

Corn and Callus Management   *81*

Cyst Removal   *53*

Depo Provera Injection   *268*

Diaphragm Fitting   *259*

Doppler Ultrasound of Lower Extremities   *153*

Ear Piercing   *118*

Electrocardiogram   *158*

Elliptical Excision and Biopsy   *43*

Enteral Tube Feeding   *190*

Epistaxis and Nasal Packing   *122*

Finger Stick Blood Glucose   *224*

Fracture Immobilization   *199*

Fungal Scraping—The KOH Test   *74*

Gastric Lavage   *174*

Ingrown Toenail Management   *88*

Nasogastric Tube Insertion and Removal   *167*

Nebulizer Treatment   *137*
Oral Airway Insertion   *146*
Papanicolaou Smear Test   *237*
Percutaneous Endoscopic Gastrostomy Tube (PEG) Management   *185*
Pessary Use   *253*
Rectal Prolapse Reduction   *181*
Reduction of Subluxed Radial Head   *218*
Removal of a Foreign Body from the Ear   *110*
Removal of a Foreign Body from the Eye   *99*
Removal of a Foreign Body from the Nose   *130*
Skin Lesion Removal   *19*
Skin Tag Removal—Cautery or Snipping   *56*
Spirometry   *139*
Splinting—Ankle Sprains   *209*
Splinting—Wrist and Hand   *202*
Subungual Hematoma Evacuation   *94*
Suturing Simple Lacerations   *28*
Tick Removal   *79*
Toenail Care in the Diabetic Patient   *84*
Treatment of Condylomata Acuminata   *247*
Treatment of Corneal Abrasion   *105*
Ulcer Debridement   *68*
Urinalysis   *9*
Urine Culture   *13*
Wart Removal—Chemical and Cryotherapy   *59*
The Wet Mount   *242*
Wound Care   *71*
X-Ray Interpretation   *221*

General Considerations for Every Procedure

Description

Description sections identify clearly the diagnostic criteria that define the problem. They help the practitioner understand the purposes behind the procedure and what constitutes a reasonable outcome.

Indications

Indications identify when this procedure is warranted, and when the problem should be referred to another provider. This should involve consideration of a complete differential diagnosis for the problem and ramifications for procedure implementation or modification based on the age of the patient.

Contraindications/Precautions

This section clearly identifies considerations that would prohibit the procedure or would cause the practitioner to proceed with extreme caution. Practitioners should make certain the patient is able to cooperate with the procedure not only by remaining quiet and not moving, but in following through with postprocedure requirements.

Patient Preparation/Education

It is mandatory to explain the procedure to every patient, without exception, and, in most cases, to have him or her, or a legal guardian, sign a consent form for the procedure.

Practitioners should always take care to provide for patient privacy and protection of modesty. In procedures requiring disrobing, adequate draping of breasts and genitalia are considered integral to establishing the proper milieu for undertaking the procedure.

Equipment

It is essential to have all the recommended equipment and to have it prepared or laid out before beginning the procedure. If materials are assembled in the order in which they are to be used, they serve as a prompt to the practitioner of the next step to take.

Procedure

Every procedure begins with the practitioner washing his or her hands. It is good practice to do this in the presence of the patient. Again, this sends the proper message to the patient about the practitioner's general standard of practice.

Assemble all resources needed before beginning the procedure. These include not only arranging the equipment, gowning, gloving, and masking of personnel as required, but assuring the presence of any assistive personnel required for the procedure.

An important part of any procedure involves cleaning equipment after the procedure and putting things away. Disposing of sharps or infectious material should follow standard agency protocol.

At the beginning of the procedure, practitioners should make certain to position the patient so that the part of the patient to be worked on is accessible. The patient should be made as comfortable as possible so that she or he will be able to remain quiet throughout the duration of the procedure. It is also very important for practitioners to find a comfortable position. Stress in standing or bending will unnecessarily tire the practitioners and make it difficult to remain focused on wh at they are doing.

The final component of the procedure should be the documentation of what has been done, the findings, and the patient's response. It is also important to record any warnings given to the patient and that the patient has been told to call back if she or he has any problems or concerns.

Postprocedure Patient Education

Explain any findings to the patient.

Provide instruction for any followup care requirements and any particular problems for which the patient should be alert. Research indicates that patients often remember only three things, and they tend to remember them in the order presented. Keep it simple.

Discuss clearly any cleaning, dressing, or medications that the patient is to use.

Always tell the patient to call or return if the problem remains, returns, or does not follow the expected postprocedure course.

Practitioner Followup/Complications

Primary care practitioners should always be alert for the development of complications, such as infections or hemorrhage. Practitioners should not hesitate to refer the patient if the postprocedure course does not proceed as usual. Remember, primary care practitioners are held responsible for whatever they accept responsibility for doing.

Pediatric Considerations

It has been said many times, but it is nonetheless true, that children are not little adults. They present a special challenge in performing both diagnostic and therapeutic procedures. Depending on their age, their behavior during any given procedure can range from frightened to ornery to docile to asleep! Even the youngest child deserves to have any questions answered and, if possible, any fears allayed.

A comforted and cooperative child is the key to success with any procedure. Parents should be utilized to the extent possible. Many procedures can be just as safely preformed with a young child seated in the mother's lap. In some situations, parents may be able to restrain a child safely and eliminate the need for frightening restraints such as papoose boards. However, the decision must be an individual one. If the parent is unduly frightened or worried about holding the child, it is wise always to err on the side of safety and utilize the appropriate restraint.

Using age-appropriate language, a procedure should always be explained to the child in advance. Young children who do not understand language can be familiarized with equipment through handling. It may be possible to mock perform the procedure on the child.

Procedures involving a developing system, such as the eye, deserve special note. The goal in care of a child is not preservation of an existing sensory system, but optimal development. Special care must always be taken to ensure that damage to an organ will not impact development. Any procedure involving the eye must be preceded by and following with visual acuity exams. Injuries involving growth plates warrant meticulous evaluation and close followup. Always remember that development is symmetrical in the young child. Vision, hearing, muscle mass, and strength should be compared side to side and differences should trigger a more thorough evaluation and, often, a referral to a subspecialist.

A final note should be made about pain management. Any practicing pediatric health professional is familiar with situations in which children are presumed to not experience pain and as a result are not provided with appropriate analgesia. Many a child has been sent home after casting of a fracture with acetaminophen as the only pain medication. In the adult population, it is well recognized that anxiety compounds pain. A child's tears may certainly begin from fear and anxiety, but many continue because of pain. It is essential to evaluate pain and treat it appropriately. The practitioner should give parents permission to contact her or him if they feel their child is experiencing an unacceptable amount of pain. The practitioner should reevaluate children who are in pain when it is no longer expected and should ask the child questions about the pain rather than relying on parents as a sole source of information. Children deserve the same level of pain relief as adults. They'll be grateful. Who knows? Maybe they'll be more cooperative next time!

Geriatric Considerations

The elderly are an extremely diverse population. Each is an unique individual and must be evaluated specifically for appropriateness of the procedure. An elective procedure should not be withheld simply because the patient is geriatric. Overall goals of care for that particular patient must be used to guide decisions about eligibility for a procedure.

The elderly are at increased risk for complications from a procedure. In general they are slower to heal and at increased risk for infection.

The presence of a dementia such as Alzheimer's disease poses special problems in completing procedures. These patients tend to have a very short attention span and may be unable to cooperate with the procedure. Their reaction to a small amount of pain or discomfort may make the procedure impossible. Attempts to restrain them usually make them more agitated. Premedicating them with a benzodiazepine such as lorazepam may help gain their cooperation.

Dermatology is an important area for special consideration in the elderly. The elderly have a large number of skin changes as a part of normal changes of aging, accelerated by exposure to the sun. Lesions suspicious for cancer should be referred to a dermatologist for biopsy. Elderly skin is susceptible to damage, slow to heal, and vulnerable to infection.

The elderly are likely to have cardiac problems and are the population in which the cardiac procedures are most utilized. One important normal change of aging is increased ectopic beats. Any arrhythmia should be properly evaluated. In doing a Holter monitor, it is important to correlate ectopy with symptoms. Interpretation of such cardiac procedures as ECGs and the Holter monitor is beyond the scope of a procedure book.

CHAPTER 1

General Laboratory Procedures

Basic Concepts of Specimen Collection

Description

   Most infectious diseases are initially suspected because of the symptoms and signs that they cause. These usually occur at the port of entry: there is a sore throat, pneumonia, diarrhea, and so on. The only way to document that an illness results from infection is to recover and identify the responsible organism. Ordinarily, this is done by drawing cultures and making a direct examination of the organism on culture media.

   Cultures may be obtained from a variety of sources: blood, bodily secretions, exudates and transudates, skin lesions, and tissue. In most cases, cultures require 24 to 48 hours to grow, but some fastidious organisms (such as mycobacteria) may require several weeks. Because of these varying requirements, it is useful to know certain technical information involved in isolating and identifying various organisms.

Indications

Specimen collection should occur whenever there is clinical suspicion of infection. However, unless there is a significant change in a patient's clinical status in a short period of time, cultures from the same site should not be repeated within 48 hours of the last set obtained.

Contraindications/Precautions

There are few, if any, contraindications to culturing a patient when clinical suspicion for infection is high. Practitioners observe several significant precautions when obtaining cultures:

- The clinical specimen must be material from the actual site of infection.
- A sufficient quantity of specimen must be obtained.
- Contamination of the culture specimen when it is obtained must be avoided. Oral flora may contaminate sputum specimens, improper cleaning of the skin may produce falsely positive blood cultures, urinary colonization may be misinterpreted as infection, and so on.
- A basic knowledge of what bacteria are considered normal flora in various body locations, as well as the proper techniques needed to obtain and interpret cultures, is fundamental in managing a patient's infection.
- Whenever possible, cultures should be obtained before initiating antibiotics.
- Culture results are influenced by such factors as number of organisms present in any given tissue, amount of specimen, host defenses, and skill of the laboratory in recovering and growing organisms.

Patient Preparation/Education

When culturing any site, practitioners should ensure that the patients understand the purpose of the culture and what they can do to assist in obtaining an uncontaminated specimen. The patients' cooperation can be increased by carefully but simply explaining what will be done to get the culture and why it is important to the patients' care.

Equipment

Equipment necessary for obtaining cultures is determined by the site of infection and type of suspected organisms. The common denominator in culturing any site is the means for sterile collection and transport of the specimen to the microbiology laboratory.

Procedure

The procedure for specimen collection varies according to site and type of culture desired, but practitioners need to follow basic principles of asepsis in every case.

Interpretation of results

Interpret culture results in light of the patient's condition, the likelihood of contamination, Gram's stain results, and associated laboratory tests. Urine cultures that are positive for more than 100,000 colony forming units (cfu) may be interpreted as being positive for infection, but if there are no white cells and leukocyte esterase is negative, the culture results are more likely to represent colonization than infection. Staph epidermitis, a normal skin organism, is more likely to be a blood culture contaminant than a pathogen.

Postprocedure patient education

Explain to the patient approximately how long it will take to get culture results back. Once the organism has been identified, it may take an additional day or two to have final antibiotic sensitivities completed. Empiric treatment may begin before the final culture results, but if sensitivities show a more effective antibiotic for the infecting bacteria, the patient's therapy may be altered.

Be certain to explain that some organisms, especially tuberculosis, require much longer than 48 hours to grow. Let patients know whether they should follow any specific precautions at home to avoid exposing other members of the household.

Practitioner Followup/Complications

Practitioners should keep aware of which patients are awaiting culture results; local medical laboratories should have preliminary results available at 48 hours. Practitioners need to follow up not only the culture results but also the sensitivity patterns of the organisms and the patient's response to therapy and make appropriate adjustments in antiinfective therapy. If in doubt, the practitioner should refer the patient to an infectious disease specialist.

Complications of cultures are primarily related to inappropriate culturing, misinterpretation of results and subsequent inappropriate therapy, and laboratory error. Any of these complications may result in increased morbidity or even mortality to the patient.

CPT BILLING CODES

87072—Culture or direct bacterial identification method, each organism, by commercial kit, any source except urine.

87075—Culture, bacterial, any source; anaerobic (isolation).

87081—Culture, bacterial, screening only, for single organisms.

87101—Culture, fungi, isolation (with or without presumptive identification); skin.

87109—Culture, mycoplasma, any source.

87118—Culture, mycobacteria, definitive identification of each organism.

86689—HTLV or HIV antibody, confirmatory test (e.g., Western Blot).

86701—HIV-1.

86792—HIV-2.

86692—Hepatitis, delta agent.

BIBLIOGRAPHY

Plorde JJ: *The diagnosis of infectious diseases.* In Wilson JD, and others, editors: *Harrison's principles of internal medicine,* ed 12, New York, 1991, McGraw-Hill.

Blood Cultures

Description

Bacteremia is the presence of bacteria in the bloodstream; it does not necessarily indicate systemic infection. Bacteremia may be transient (as in cellulitis or abscess), intermittent (an undrained abdominal abscess), or continuous (intravascular infections such as infective endocarditis). *Septicemia* is a general term for any microorganism in the bloodstream. Septicemia occurs when circulating microorganisms multiply at a rate that exceeds the body's ability to phagocytize the organisms. Detection of bacteremia and fungemia by clinicians is of primary importance in reducing the morbidity and mortality associated with septicemia. Primary care practitioners must be aware of the indications for drawing blood cultures, the interpretation of culture results, and the appropriate therapy for these results.

Indications

Blood cultures should be obtained if there is clinical suspicion of septicemia. (Acutely ill patients and those with evidence of hemodynamic decompensation should be referred for possible hospital admission.)

A patient who presents with a complaint of easy fatiguability, fever, chills, tachycardia, and hyperventilation in the absence of other identifiable cause should have blood cultures made.

Patients at risk for bacteremia are those who have been hospitalized or are immunocompromised (cancer, HIV, lupus, diabetes).

Patients who have not responded to treatment with appropriate antibiotics for documented infections need to have the blood culture procedure repeated.

Contraindications/Precautions

There are no absolute contraindications for drawing blood cultures. Great care must be used in preparing venipuncture sites to decrease the risk of contamination by normal skin flora. Femoral sites are not recommended secondary to high bacterial colony counts in that area.

Blood cultures take time. Although initial reports may be available within 24 to 48 hours, some organisms require 5 to 7 days before reading. Some microorganisms grow poorly in conventional culture media and may require special culture bottles.

Practitioners should refer acutely ill patients to a physician.

Patient Preparation/Education

Before the procedure, practitioners should explain the purpose of obtaining the blood culture to the patient. It should be emphasized that often culture results may be known within 24 to 48 hours, but in some cases it will take longer. The patient should continue to monitor his or her own temperature. If antibiotics are ordered, they should be continued as prescribed. The patient should be advised to call for the results of the culture after 48 hours if he or she has not already been contacted.

Equipment

- Gloves
- Two 10-cc syringes
- Four 20-gauge needles
- Two sets of blood culture bottles (aerobic and anaerobic bottle in each set)
- Identification labels
- Isopropyl alcohol
- Povidone–iodine solution (Betadine)
- Needle disposal box
- Tourniquet

Procedure

1. Locate a suitable vein and apply the tourniquet with sufficient pressure to prevent venous return.

2. Don gloves.
3. Clean the skin first with alcohol and then with iodine–povidone solution (if the patient is not allergic to iodine).
4. Insert the needle and aspirate 10 to 20 ml of blood. Failure to inoculate culture media with enough blood may result in a false-negative culture report.
5. Release the tourniquet.
6. Clean the rubber diaphragm of the blood culture bottle with alcohol only (Betadine solution may interfere with the automatic processing of some culture collection systems).
7. Change the needle on the syringe; first inject anaerobic bottle with 5 to 10 ml of blood to prevent introduction of air into the bottle.
8. Repeat the blood drawing procedure for a second set of cultures 15 to 20 minutes following the first set.
9. Label each bottle with the patient's name, the date and time the specimen has been drawn, and the site.

Interpretation of results

Interpretation of blood culture results should take into account the concentration of organisms, the technique used in obtaining the cultures, and the length of time for the culture to become positive. Not all positive blood cultures are clinically significant. Contaminated cultures, which typically grow *Staphylococcus epidermidis*, *Corynebacterium*, and other "skin flora," may mistakenly be interpreted as positive cultures. False-positive cultures typically grow more slowly than true-positive cultures and repeat cultures are rarely positive for the same organism.

Lack of blood culture growth does not necessarily indicate sterile blood. The concentration of organisms, or the inoculum, in the blood may be relatively low, or the organism may not grow well enough in standard culture media to be identified. Interpret all blood culture results cautiously and in the context of the patient's clinical picture.

Postprocedure patient education

Instruct the patient to observe venipuncture sites for bleeding or purulent drainage.

Some bruising at the site of blood drawing may be normal.

Instruct the patient to notify the practitioner if fever, chills, shaking, nausea, or vomiting occur or recur.

Practitioner Followup/Complications

Blood culture results should be checked at 24 and 48 hours.

Most labs will hold blood culture for 5 to 7 days before issuing a final report.

Once a definitive identification is made, most labs will also run a sensitivity panel. It is crucial to place the patient on the correct antibiotic for the identified organism.

Practitioners who are unfamiliar with how to read a sensitivity panel should refer the patient to an infectious disease specialist.

CPT BILLING CODES

87040—Culture, bacterial, definitive; blood (includes anaerobic screen).

87103—Culture, fungi, isolation (with or without presumptive identification); blood.

BIBLIOGRAPHY

Smith-Elekes S, Weinstein MP: Blood cultures, *Infect Dis Clin North Am,* 7(2):221, 1993.

Washington JA: Bacteria, fungi, and parasites. In Mandell GL, Douglas RG Jr, Bennett JE, editors: *Principles and practice of infectious diseases,* ed 3, New York, 1990, Churchill Livingstone.

Urinalysis

Description

Urinalysis is an examination of the urine that consists of three components: (A) physical examination of the urine, i.e., color, turbidity; (B) chemical examination of the urine, i.e., pH, glucose, ketones, etc.; and (C) microscopic examination of the urine.

Indications

Urinalysis is performed to obtain information for screening and diagnosis and monitoring of disease states.

It is an inexpensive way to test large numbers of people for renal disease, urinary bladder disease, and asymptomatic development of conditions such as diabetes mellitus and liver disease.

During pregnancy, urinalysis is used frequently to screen for metabolic disorders such as diabetes and the proteinuria associated with preeclampsia.

Contraindications/Precautions

The collection of urine and performance of urinalysis is a safe procedure with no risk to the patient. The practitioner must be aware of conditions, chemicals, and drugs that may interfere with the accuracy of the analysis.

Patient Preparation/Education

In outpatient settings the patient usually collects the specimen but a nurse or laboratory technician may assist. Explanation of the correct procedure is vital because the accuracy of the laboratory analysis depends upon the quality of the specimen.

If a woman patient is menstruating or has a heavy vaginal discharge, she should insert a vaginal tampon before collecting the specimen.

Equipment

To collect a midstream specimen, which is commonly used for routine urinalysis, the practitioner should assemble the following equipment.

- Clear, disposable, plastic container of a 6- to 10-oz capacity. It should be chemically clean for urinalysis only and sterile if a culture may be indicated.
- Two to three perineal wipes.

- Equipment for hand washing.
- Written patient instructions for specimen collection.
- Label for the container.

SPECIMEN FOR PHYSICAL EXAMINATION
- Clear plastic container
- White background against which to observe urine
- Urinometer or refractometer for specific gravity or chemical specific gravity tapes (such as spG tapes)

SPECIMEN FOR CHEMICAL EXAMINATION
- Reagent strip
- Manufacturer's color chart

SPECIMEN FOR MICROSCOPIC EXAMINATION
- Centrifuge
- Centrifuge tube
- Dropper/pipette
- Glass slide and cover slide
- Microscope
- Nonsterile gloves

SPECIMEN FOR CULTURE
- See urine culture procedure

Procedure

Instruct the patient as follows:

1. Wash hands.
2. Open the specimen container, placing the lid sterile side up on the counter.
3. *Female:* Stand over toilet, use one hand to separate the labia, wipe the area of the meatus two to three times, wiping front to back once with each wipe.
   Male: Stand over toilet, hold penis with one hand, wipe two or three times around the urinary meatus once with each wipe.

4. Urinate first into the toilet, then into the specimen cup, and finish urinating into the toilet. The container does not need to be full, but it should contain at least ¼ cup to allow adequate testing.

5. Do not touch the inside of the container and only touch the outside of the lid.

6. Screw the lid tightly on the container; label with the patient's name and the date and deliver it to the collection area or person.

7. The specimen should be examined within 1 hour after collection. (After 1 hour, multiple changes occur in urine, rendering the analysis inaccurate). A specimen that cannot be examined within 1 hour may be refrigerated for up to 24 hours; the specimen should be allowed to return to room temperature before examination.

Physical examination

Note: It is best to pour the urine into the centrifuge tube before the urinalysis is performed; then the urine left in the specimen container may be used for culture if necessary.

1. Determine appearance: Hold the urine up to the light, against a white background, to examine for the presence of turbidity and to note the color. Terms used to describe turbidity include clear, hazy, slightly cloudy, cloudy, turbid, and milky.

2. Specific gravity: For refractometer, place 1 or 2 drops of urine on the prism, focus the instrument with a good light source, and take the reading directly from the specific gravity (spG) scale.

Chemical examination

1. Mix the specimen well, then dip the reagent strip completely, but briefly, into the specimen.

2. Remove excess urine when you withdraw the strip from specimen by tapping the strip against the inside of the container.

3. Hold the strip horizontal when comparing it to the color chart to prevent mixing of reagents.

4. Follow the manufacturer's directions for each type of reagent to determine the number of seconds required for measurement. Compare the strip against the color chart on the container. When precise timing cannot be performed, most manufacturers suggest reading at 60 seconds, but never later than 120 seconds.

Microscopic examination

1. Examine the urine while it is fresh.
2. Centrifuge 10 ml of urine for 5 minutes at a centrifugal force of 400 in a specially identified specimen tube.
3. Using a pipette, remove 9 ml of the supernate (clear fluid) and resuspend the sediment in the remaining 1 ml.
4. Take 1 drop of the resuspended sediment and transfer it to a microscope slide; put a cover slip over the slide.
5. Examine the slide first under low power, reading at least 10 low-power fields (lpf), scanning to evaluate what is on the slide and counting and averaging the number of casts, if any, that are found.
6. Examine 10 high-power fields (hpf) and count the cells; report the average number per field.
7. Reporting may vary among laboratories. Red blood cells, white blood cells, epithelial cells, and crystals are usually reported as number per hpf. Casts are listed as number per lpf. Other elements are listed as rare, few, many, and packed. The term "too numerous to count" (TNTC) may be used when markedly increased numbers of cells and crystals are seen. Casts, epithelial cells, and crystals must also be identified as to their type.

Postprocedure patient education

Explanations to the patient after the procedure depend primarily on the purpose of the urinalysis (screening, diagnostic, monitoring), the results, and the plan of care.

Practitioner Followup/Complications

Additional tests may need to be ordered to clarify the diagnosis if abnormalities are found. Findings should be documented.

CPT BILLING CODES

81002—Urinalysis, without microscopy, nonautomated.

81007—Urinalysis, bacteriuria screen, by nonculture technique, commercial kit.

81015—Urinalysis, microscopic only.

BIBLIOGRAPHY

Ross LD, Neely AE: *Textbook of urinalysis and body fluids,* East Norwalk, Conn, 1983, Appleton-Century-Crofts.

Strasinger SK: *Urinalysis and body fluids: a self-instructional text,* Philadelphia, 1989, FA Davis.

Urine under the microscope, Nutley, NJ, 1978, Hoffmann-LaRouche.

Urine Culture

Description

Urinary tract infections are common among the primary care patient population. Traditional diagnosis and treatment regimens for acute cystitis have been estimated to cost $140 per episode. Untreated, an uncomplicated urinary tract infection (UTI) can progress to more complicated problems, including kidney infections.

Early diagnosis and treatment of UTIs can reduce the morbidity and cost associated with these infections. Urinary infections are frequently divided into lower UTI, or cystitis, and upper UTI, acute pyelonephritis.

Indications

One of the cardinal symptoms of any UTI is dysuria. Other symptoms include frequency, urgency, burning, nocturia, incontinence, and suprapubic or pelvic pain.

Differential diagnosis of UTI must include other inflammatory or infectious problems, such as sexually transmitted diseases, vaginitis, or obstructive disorders (Table 1-1).

Contraindications/Precautions

A major problem in collecting urine for cultures arises when there is contamination with vaginal or labial bacteria. Catheteriza-

Table 1-1

Differential Diagnosis of Dysuria Syndromes

| | Dysuria | | Onset | | History | | | |
	Internal	External	Acute	Subacute	Vaginal discharge or odor, pruritus, external lesions	New SP, multiple SPs, SP with STD	Frequency, urgency, hematuria, suprapubic pain, diaphragm use	Fever, chills, sweats, nausea, vomiting
Acute pyelonephritis	+/-	-	+	-	-	-	+/-	+
Acute cystitis	+	-	+	-	-	-	+	-
Urethritis caused by STD								
HSV	+	+/-	-	+	+	+	+/-	-
GC	+	-	+	-	+	+	+/-	-
CT	+	-	-	+	+	+	+/-	-
Vulvovaginitis (bacterial vaginosis, trichomoniasis, yeast, genital HSV)	-	+	-	+	+	+	-	-
Noninflammatory dysuria (trauma, irritant, allergy)	?	?	?	?	-	?	-	-

	Physical examination			Laboratory				
	Vaginal or cervical discharge, vulvar lesions	Suprapubic tenderness	Flank tenderness, fever	Abnormal vaginal fluid or cervical smear	Culture of genital lesions, cervix, or urethra positive for CT, CC, HSV	Pyuria	Microscopic hematuria or bacteriuria	Urine culture (>10² cfu/ml)
Acute pyelonephritis	–	+/–	+	–	–	+	+	+
Acute cystitis	–	+/–	–	–	–	+	+/–	+
Urethritis caused by STD								
HSV	+	–	–	+/–	+	+	–	–
GC	+	–	–	+	+	+	–	–
CT	+	–	–	+	+	+	–	–
Vulvovaginitis (bacterial vaginosis, trichomoniasis, yeast, genital HSV)	+	–	–	+	+/–	–	–	–
Noninflammatory dysuria (trauma, irritant, allergy)	–	–	–	–	–	–	–	–

SOURCE: Johnson JR, Stamm WE, Diagnosis and treatment of acute urinary tract infections, *Infect Dis Clin North Am* 1(4):776-777, 1987.
ABBREVIATIONS: STD = sexually transmitted disease; SP = sex partner; CT = *Chlamydia trachomatis*; GC = *N. gonorrhoeae*; HSV = herpes simplex.

tion is one way to solve this problem; however, in most primary care settings, this may not be feasible. Catheterization of a patient with acute cystitis may predispose susceptible individuals to bacteremia and subsequent endocarditis. The risk of such a serious complication is fortunately very small.

Patient Preparation/Education

Explain urine collection procedures to the patient.

Emphasize the importance of not contaminating the specimen with skin flora from the patient's fingers, labia, or foreskin.

Equipment

- Sterile specimen container with tight-fitting (screw-on) lid
- Cleansing towelettes
- Soap and water

Procedure

In the outpatient setting, a "midstream" voided specimen is the most practical way to obtain urine. Instruct the patient to do the following:

1. Wash the hands and open the container.
2. *Female:* Using the index and middle fingers of the nondominant hand, spread the labia and wipe perineal area from front to back. Without allowing the labia to meet, repeat the wiping two more times. If vaginal discharge or menses are present, a tampon should first be inserted.
   Male: Retract the foreskin and, using the cleansing swab or towelette, clean end of penis using a circular motion moving from meatus outward.
3. Initiate the urine stream.
4. After a single stream is achieved, pass the specimen container into the stream and obtain the sample.

5. Remove the container before the flow of urine stops and before releasing the labia or penis. This decreases the risk of contaminating the specimen with skin flora.
6. Replace the cap on the container and wipe off the outside of the container.
7. Wash the hands again.
8. Label the specimen container with the patient's name, the date, and the time of collection.
9. The specimen should reach the laboratory within 30 minutes of collection.

Interpretation of results

Evaluate urine cultures in conjunction with other documentation that confirms infection. The presence of bacteria alone does not make a diagnosis of UTI. Many older women have asymptomatic bacteriuria.

Microscopic evaluation and the presence of white blood cells is essential to confirm infection. Testing for the presence of leukocyte esterase by dipstick is a relatively reliable method for determining the presence of white blood cells in the urine. The sensitivity of dipstick tests diminishes when bacterial counts of less than 10,000 colonies per milliliter are present.

Postprocedure patient education

Explain to the patient that urine culture results will be available within 24 to 48 hours.

Explain that empiric antibiotic therapy will be initiated before final culture results are available. Should the culture reveal resistant organisms, antibiotic therapy will be adjusted.

New onset of fever, shaking chills, headache, nausea, or vomiting should be reported immediately.

Practitioner Followup/Complications

Posttherapy cultures should be obtained only in those patients who have a history of frequent UTI's, drug-resistant organisms, or persistent symptoms. In these instances, posttreatment cultures should be obtained 7 to 14 days after therapy.

Complications of UTI can be serious. Inflammation of the renal parenchyma and pelvis may lead to acute pyelonephritis and possibly to bacteremia.

CPT BILLING CODES

81002—Urinalysis, without microscopy, nonautomated.

81007—Bacteriuria screen, by nonculture technique, commercial kit.

81015—Urinalysis, microscopic only.

87086—Culture, bacterial, urine; quantitative, colony count.

BIBLIOGRAPHY

Boscia JA, Kaye D: Asymptomatic bacteriuria in the elderly, *Infect Dis Clin North Am* 1(4):893, 1987.
Culhane JK: Clinical uses of the leukocyte esterase test, *Primary Care* 13(4):679, 1986.
Johnson JR, Stamm WE: Diagnosis and treatment of acute urinary tract infections, *Infect Dis Clin North Am* 4:773, 1987.

CHAPTER 2

Dermatologic Procedures

Skin Lesion Removal

There are many different approaches to treating lesions; the decision of which one to use is a clinical judgment. The decision should be based on the type, location, and size of the lesion; the possibility of malignancy; and practitioner preference. Carcinoma is very common, especially in older patients. If there is any chance of carcinoma, the practitioner should either do a full excision with biopsy or refer to a dermatologist. The practitioner should biopsy any nonhealing, changing, or enlarging skin lesion. Virtually all lesions that are excised should be sent for biopsy unless the diagnosis is absolutely certain. If using elliptical excision, the practitioner should remove the entire lesion including the lesion margins. Referral may be necessary if the lesion is deep. Lesions on the face should be referred to a specialist if an acceptable cosmetic result is important.

Many of the benign lesions, such as skin tags, need only be removed for cosmetic or practical reasons such as clothing rubbing on the lesion and causing discomfort.

The following box provides practitioners with management options for the more common lesions they may see in their practice.

Skin lesion	Treatment
Simple laceration	Suture, Steri-Strip
Skin tag	Snip, cautery
Suspicious lesion	Excisional biopsy
Sebaceous (epidermal) cyst	Cyst removal, incision and drainage
Common wart	Chemical treatment, cryotherapy
Plantar wart	Cryotherapy, chemical treatment
Seborrheic keratosis	Excisional biopsy
Abscess	Incision and drainage

Anesthesia–Local, Topical, and Digital Nerve Block

Description

Anesthesia is indicated for many of the procedures discussed in this book. Local, topical, and peripheral nerve block anesthesia can be used by the practitioner to provide patient comfort and cooperation during the procedure. Topical anesthesia utilizes various preparations placed on the tissue needing anesthesia without the use of a needle. Local anesthesia is injected at the site where anesthesia is desired. In peripheral nerve blocks, anesthesia is injected to block primary neuropathways, resulting in temporary interruption of conduction of nerve pain impulses while the patient remains awake. The type of anesthesia used depends on a variety of factors: the size and location of the wound, the presence of infection, the blood supply to the area, and the patient's pain threshold and ability to cooperate with the procedure.

Indications

The purpose is to provide local, effective, and fast anesthesia to allow other minor procedures to be accomplished with minimal pain to the patient.

Topical anesthesia is used in the treatment of superficial lesions and on patients who have a phobia of needles. This is especially useful for children. Topical anesthesia is also useful to decrease the pain of local anesthesia or nerve block. TAC (see Equipment) is used for scalp and facial laceration repair. EMLA cream (see Equipment) under occlusion on intact skin is used for suture removal and for painful injections in children. Ice or ethyl chloride is used for skin tag clipping and abscess incision and drainage.

Local anesthesia is used for most minor procedures such as suturing.

Digital nerve blocks are used in common minor surgical or orthopedic procedures of the fingers and toes.

Contraindications/Precautions

Patients need to be assessed for allergies to anesthesia products. The two groups of anesthetics do not cross react, so patients who report an allergy to procaine (Novocaine) or tetracaine can use lidocaine (Xylocaine), mepivacaine (Carbocaine), or bupivacaine (Marcaine) without inducing an allergic response.

Some patients may be allergic to the preservative in multidose bottles. These patients require single-dose vials.

Use of a vasoconstrictor such as epinephrine is contraindicated on the extremities; vasoconstrictors need to be used with extreme care in areas where vasoconstriction could be a problem. Use epinephrine with caution in patients with peripheral vascular disease, diabetes, or heart disease. Do not use epinephrine in an infected wound.

Practitioners should not attempt anesthesia if substantial tissue damage and bleeding exist.

Patient Preparation/Education

Practitioners should explain that the procedure will stop the patient's pain.

Practitioners need to explain the importance of the patient's not moving during the procedure.

Equipment

TOPICAL ANESTHESIA
- Topical anesthetic—see Table 2-1.
- TAC (tetracaine 2.5 mg; adrenaline 1:1000, 2.5 cc; cocaine 0.59 g; dissolved in sufficient sterile water to make 5 cc) and sterile cotton balls.
- EMLA (eutectic mixture of local anesthetic) and occlusive dressing.

LOCAL ANESTHESIA
- Sodium bicarbonate (Neutra-caine) 7.5%, 5-ml vial
- One 18-gauge needle to draw up solution
- One 27- to 30-gauge, 1-inch length needle for injection
- Alcohol swabs
- Appropriate size syringe (2 to 10 cc)
- Anesthetic of choice (see Tables 2-2 and 2-3 and the box for selection)

PERIPHERAL NERVE BLOCK
- Sterile field
- Betadine
- Ethyl chloride
- Local anesthetic agent (lidocaine)
- One 18-gauge needle to draw up solution
- One 25- to 30-gauge needle for injection
- Appropriate size syringe (2 to 10 cc)
- Sterile gloves

Procedure

Topical anesthesia
1. Apply cotton balls soaked in TAC to a wound on the scalp or face for 10 minutes.
2. Apply EMLA to intact skin and apply an occlusive dressing 30 to 90 minutes before the procedure.
3. Rub the skin with ice for 10 seconds; anesthesia lasts 2 seconds.

Table 2-1

Topical Anesthetic Preparations

Anesthetic	Concentration (%)	Form	Tissue
Benzocaine	1-5	Cream	Skin and mucous membrane
	20	Ointment	Skin and mucous membrane
	20	Aerosol	Skin and mucous membrane
Cocaine	4	Solution	Ear, nose, throat
Dibucaine	0.25-1	Cream	Skin
	0.25-1	Ointment	Skin
	0.25-1	Aerosol	Skin
	0.25	Solution	Ear
	2.5	Suppository	Rectum
Cyclonine	0.5-1	Solution	Skin, oropharynx, tracheobronchial tree, urethra, rectum
Lidocaine	2-4	Solution	Oropharynx, tracheobronchial tree, nose
	2	Jelly	Urethra
	2.5-5	Ointment	Skin, mucous membrane, rectum
	2	Viscous solution	Oropharynx
	10	Suppository	Rectum
	10	Aerosol	Gingival mucosa
Tetracaine	0.5-1	Ointment	Skin, rectum, mucous membrane
	0.5-1	Cream	Skin, rectum, mucous membrane
	0.25-1	Solution	Nose, tracheobronchial tree

From Pfenninger JL, Fowler GC: *Procedures for primary care physicians*, St Louis, 1994, Mosby; MODIFIED FROM Covino BG, Vassallo HG: *Local anesthetics: mechanisms of action and clinical use*, New York, 1976, Grune & Stratton.

Table 2-2

Commonly Used Local Anesthetics in the Office Setting

Local anesthetic	Onset (min)	Duration (hr)	Equivalent conc. (%)
Lidocaine (Xylocaine)	1	0.5-1	1
Lidocaine w/epinephrine	1	2-6	1
Mepivacaine (Carbocaine)	3-5	0.75-1.5	1
Dibucaine (Nupercaine)	15	3-4	0.25
Dibucaine w/epinephrine	15	6	0.25
Bupivacaine (Marcaine)	5	2-4	0.25
Bupivacaine w/epinephrine	5	3-7	0.25
Etidocaine (Duranest)	3-5	3-7	0.5

From Pfenninger JL, Fowler GC: *Procedures for primary care physicians,* St Louis, 1994, Mosby; MODIFIED FROM Olin BR, editor: *Drug facts and comparisons,* St Louis, 1993, Mosby.

Table 2-3

Maximum Dosages of Commonly Used Local Anesthetics

Anesthetic	Concentration	Maximum dose
Lidocaine (Xylocaine)	1%	4.5 mg/kg not to exceed 300 mg (30 cc in adult)
Lidocaine (Xylocaine) w/epinephrine	1%	7 mg/kg not to exceed 500 mg (50 cc in adult)
Bupivacaine (Marcaine)	0.25%	3 mg/kg not to exceed 175 mg (50 cc per average adult)
Bupivacaine (Marcaine) w/epinephrine	0.25%	3 mg/kg not to exceed 225 mg

From Pfenninger JL, Fowler GC: *Procedures for primary care physicians,* St Louis, 1994, Mosby.

Selection of Local Anesthetics/Effects

Lidocaine (Xylocaine) without epinephrine

Can cause vasodilatation.
0.5 to 1 hour duration depending on site/vascularity.
Use in contaminated wounds.
Use in fingers, nose, penis, toes, earlobes.
Use if vascular disease is present or if patient is immunocompromised.
Use if there are cerebrovascular or cardiovascular risks.
Use for nerve blocks.

Lidocaine (Xylocaine) with epinephrine

Causes vasoconstriction.
Has longer duration.
Use in highly vascular areas to improve visualization of field.
Use in clean wounds.
In general, do not use on fingers, nose, penis, toes, and earlobes.

Bupivacaine (Marcaine)

For longer duration.
For nerve blocks.

FROM Pfenninger JL, Fowler GC: *Procedures for primary care physicians,* St Louis, 1994, Mosby.

4. Spray site with ethyl chloride for 1 to 2 seconds; anesthesia lasts 2 seconds.

Local anesthesia

1. Add 1 ml of a 1 mg/ml sodium bicarbonate solution to 10 cc of a 1% concentration of anesthetic to eliminate burning on injection. Buffered lidocaine is stable for 1 week at room temperature and 10 days if refrigerated.
2. Draw up the anesthetic with the 18-gauge needle into the syringe. Between 1 and 10 cc of anesthetic will be used depending on the size and location of the area to be anesthetized.
3. Change the needle to the one to be used for injection.
4. Inject the anesthetic intradermally or subcutaneously. Insert the

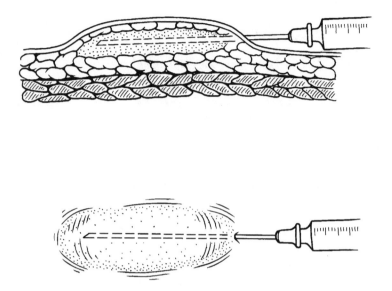

Fig. 2-1 Subcutaneous infiltration. Injection is made during advance and withdrawal of the needle.

needle and aspirate to check for blood return before administering anesthetic. Subcutaneous injection will take longer than intradermal injection to take effect. With the needle parallel to the skin, inject anesthetic as you advance and withdraw the needle through the area to be infiltrated (Fig. 2-1).

5. Wait for the local anesthetic to work before beginning the procedure. Test for sensation before proceeding.

Peripheral nerve block

1. Draw up the syringe with anesthesia. Satisfactory anesthesia should be possible with 2.5 cc of lidocaine 2%. This avoids complete vascular compression by the increased pressure from injected local anesthetic.
2. Administer ethyl chloride to numb the skin.
3. Select a site proximal to the dorsal digital nerve.
4. Aspirate for blood return then administer approximately 0.5 cc 2% Lidocaine (Fig. 2-2).
5. Advance the needle at a 90-degree angle toward the plantar digital nerve. The needle may be palpated with support from an index finger under the plantar surface.

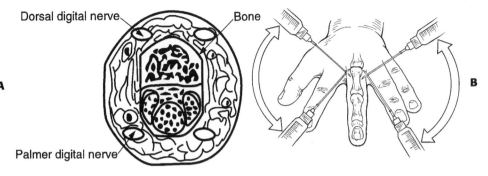

Fig. 2-2 Anatomy and injection technique for digital nerve block. **A** Four digital nerves of the finger. The bone is used as a landmark to find the proper plane of the dorsal digital nerve. **B** Digital nerve block of the finger. The sites of the nerves are injected bilaterally. To obtain the optimal effect, after blocking the nerves, place a "ring" of anesthetic entirely around the digit close to the bone. Inject superiorly over the bone and inferiorly under the bone in the subcutaneous plane. (**B** from Trott A: *Wounds and lacerations: emergency care and closure,* ed 2, St Louis, 1991, Mosby. Used with permission.)

6. Withdraw the needle proximally 2 mm, aspirate for blood return, and inject approximately 0.5 cc 2% lidocaine.
7. Repeat the identical procedure to the opposite side of the hallux.

Test for loss of sensation before proceeding with the surgery (approximately 3 to 5 minutes).

Postprocedure patient education

Explain any postprocedure instructions for care.

Postprocedure pain management should depend upon the extent of the injury.

Practitioner Followup/Complications

Allergy to lidocaine is rare but present.

CPT BILLING CODE

The CPT code will depend on the surgical procedure being performed after anesthesia; there is no single code for digital nerve block.

BIBLIOGRAPHY

Ernst AA, and others: 1% lidocaine versus 0.5% diphenhydramine for local anesthesia in minor laceration repair, *Ann Emerg Med* 23(6):1328, 1994.

Ferrera PC, Chandler R: Anesthesia in the emergency setting: Part I. Hand and foot injuries, *Am Fam Physician* 50(3):569, 1994.

Ferrera PC, Chandler R: Anesthesia in the emergency setting: Part II. Head and neck, eye and rib injuries, *Am Fam Physician* 50(4):797, 1994.

Joyce TH: Topical anesthesia and pain management before venipuncture, *J Pediatr* 122(5, Pt 2):S24, 1993.

Pfenninger JL, Fowler GC: *Procedures for primary care physicians,* St Louis, 1994, Mosby.

Rivellini D: Local and regional anesthesia. Nursing implications, *Nurs Clin North Am* 28(3):547, 1993.

Roberts PW: *Useful procedures in medical practice,* Philadelphia, 1986, Lea & Febiger.

Suturing Simple Lacerations

Description

In suturing the simple laceration, practitioners approximate the wound edges so that the wound can heal without infection and with minimal scarring. Sutures are threads or wire used to sew the body tissues together. Proper wound closure is done with minimal trauma and tension to the tissues to control bleeding. When the tissue planes are being brought together, it is important to obliterate dead space, provide hemostasis where ligatures have been used, approximate deep layers, and unite the skin margins. Dead space allows for the accumulation of blood or serum, which acts as a natural culture medium for organisms causing wound infection.

Indications

Wounds need to be closed to allow cessation of bleeding, prevent infection, preserve function, and restore appearance.

The wound should be closed within 4 to 8 hours after the injury. Waiting longer increases the risk of infection. In some cases, a delay of up to 24 hours is acceptable.

If the laceration is not deep and edges are easily approximated, steri-strips rather than sutures may be used as long as there is no tension or pressure on the area.

Contraindications/Precautions

Practitioners refer the following types of wounds to specialists: wounds in which there is damage to the blood supply, the nerves, or the joint; wounds on the face; or wounds that have tissue damage or infection.

Patients with special medical problems, such as diabetes, uremia, hypoxia, circulatory impairment, hypertrophic scarring/keloid history, or immunosuppression, that may interfere with wound healing should have special consideration.

The elderly have delayed healing of skin wounds and are at increased risk for infections.

Precaution must also be taken when administering anesthesia to patients with hypertension, liver impairment, malignant hyperthermia, and diabetes. (See Procedure on anesthesia.)

It is important that the sutures be completely removed in a timely manner. Fragments left in the wound can act as a foreign body and cause complications such as infection.

Patient Preparation/Education

The practitioner reassures the patient.

The practitioner administers a tetanus injection if necessary (see box).

The practitioner gives immunoglobulin 250 U IM for a moderate wound, 500 U IM for a severe wound as indicated below.

The practitioner gives a Td booster 0.5 ml IM as indicated below. Do not give pertussis over the age of 7.

Tetanus Prophylaxis			
	Last Td/DPT		
Wound	**Not immunized**	**5-10 years**	**10 yr+**
Clean	Td or DPT	None	Td
Dirty	Ig + Td/DPT	Td	Td + Ig

*DPT, Primary series for children; *Td*, tetanus plus a small amount of diptheria used to elicit memory response in adults—not given to children; *Ig*, immunoglobulin.

Children younger than 7 years old should get DPT if they are unimmunized or have not completed their primary series. DT is given to children under age 7 who have had an adverse reaction to primary DPT series.

Equipment

- Basic suture tray, which usually contains: Webster needle holder, iris scissors, Adson forceps with teeth, curved mosquito hemostat, 4 × 4 gauze sponges, sterile fenestrated paper drapes.
- Suture material (for selection, see box below)
- Needle (for selection, see box below)
- Sterile normal saline, and Betadine

Suture Selection

Choose sutures based on their basic characteristics of tissue reactivity, knot holding, wick action, tensile strength, and cost. (See Table 2-4 for suture selection.) Suture material also can be absorbable or nonabsorbable and either monofilament or braided. The size of the sutures and the needle type are also to be considered.

Tissue reactivity is an important consideration in selecting suture material. High tissue reactivity may lead to scar and fissure formation.

Knots are the weakest part of the suture. Proper knotting technique is essential. The different suture materials vary in their knot holding properties.

Only nonabsorbable sutures are required for suturing superficial lacerations. Absorbable sutures are used for layered closure of deep lacerations.

Braided suture is stronger and holds knots better than monofilament. Monofilament is less likely to harbor infection.

Suture size is indicated by 0. More 0's designate smaller sized sutures. For example, 4-0 is smaller than 3-0 suture material. Smaller sutures leave less of a scar but are not as strong as larger sutures. (See Tables 2-4 and 2-5 for suture selection and use.)

Table 2-4

Common Suture Materials

Suture	Types	Makeup	Use	Tissue reaction	Absorption rate	Tensile strength retention
Absorbable						
Gut	Plain	Mammalian collagen	Superficial vessels and quick healing subcutaneous tissues	Moderate	70 days	7 to 10 days
Gut	Chromic	Mammalian collagen	Versatile; also good in the presence of infection; do not use on skin because of reaction	Moderate	90 days	21 to 28 days
Polyglycolic acid (Dexon*)	Mono	Synthetic polymer	Buried sutures; good tensile and knot strength	Mild	40% 7 days	20% in 15 days 5% in 28 days
Polydioxanone (PDS†)	Mono	Polyester polymer	Versatile; body cavity closure, bowel	Mild	210 days	70% in 14 days 50% in 28 days
Polyglactic acid (Vicryl†)	Braided	Coated polymer	Subcutaneous skin; buried sutures	Mild	60 to 90 days	60% in 14 days 30% in 21 days
Polyglyconate (Maxon)	Mono	Polyester	Smoother knot and excellent first-throw holding	Mild	180 to 210 days	81% in 14 days 59% in 28 days

Continued.

FROM Pfenninger JL, Fowler GC: *Procedures for primary care physicians*, St Louis, 1994, Mosby.
*Dexon Plus has a synthetic coating to facilitate knot tying and passage through tissue.
†Vicryl, Prolene, and PDS are registered trademarks of Ethicon, Inc.

Table 2-4—cont'd

Common Suture Materials—cont'd

Suture	Types	Makeup	Use	Tissue reaction	Absorption rate	Tensile strength retention
Nonabsorbable						
Cotton	Twisted fibers	Cotton fiber	Ligating, some skin but generally too reactive	Minimal	Never; encapsulated in the body	50% in 6 months 30% in 2 years
Silk	Braided	Silkworm spun fiber	Ligating, some skin but rarely used	Moderate	2 years	Gone in one year
Steel	Mono	Alloy Fe-Ni-Cr	Tendons, sternum, abdominal wall	Low	Never; encapsulated in the body	Indefinite
Nylon (Ethilon, Dermalon)	Mono	Synthetic polymer	Skin	Very low	20% a year	Loses 20% a year
Polyester (Mersilene)	Braided	Polyester	Cardiovascular, general, and plastic surgery	Minimal	Never; encapsulated in the body	Indefinite
Polypropylene (Prolene†)	Mono	Synthetic polymer	Skin, vascular, plastic surgery	Minimal	Never; encapsulated in the body	Indefinite

Table 2-5

Common Suture Use

	Skin (interrupted)	Skin (subcuticular)	Buried	Removal
Face	5-0 or 6-0 nylon	4-0 or 5-0 Prolene	4-0 or 5-0 synthetic absorbable or 6-0 clear nylon	4 to 7 days
Extremities, trunk	4-0 or 5-0 nylon	3-0 or 4-0 synthetic absorbable	4-0 Prolene or 3-0 or 4-0 synthetic absorbable	7 to 14 days

FROM Pfenninger JL, Fowler GC: *Procedures for primary care physicians,* St Louis, 1994, Mosby.

Needle Selection

Use a cutting needle for suturing skin. A three-eights curvature is usually adequate. The manufacturers have codes for their products denoting purpose and size. "For skin" (FS) and "cutting" (CE) needles should be used on thick skin. On cosmetic areas, plastic (P), plastic skin (PS), premium (PRE), or precision cosmetic (PC) needles are recommended. Facial closures are often done with a P-3 needle, whereas other areas with thicker skin require an FS-2 or FS-3 (Figs. 2-3 and 2-4).

- A 60- to 30-cc syringe and an 18-gauge needle, or irrigating device
- Sterile gloves, mask, and eye protection
- Anesthetizing agent (see procedure on anesthesia)

For suture removal

- Fine scissors
- Clamps or pickups
- Bandage
- Gloves
- Other—Determine whether steri-strips will be necessary or further wound care interventions needed.

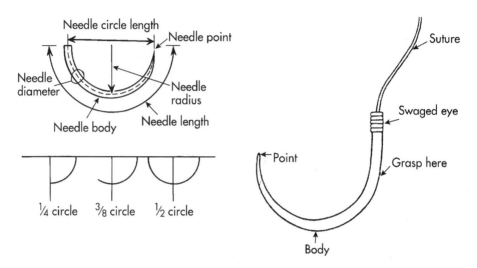

Fig. 2-3 Anatomy of a surgical needle. (From Pfenninger JL, Fowler GC: *Procedures for primary care physicians,* St Louis, 1994, Mosby.)

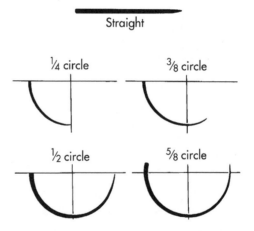

Fig. 2-4 Needle body shapes. (From Pfenninger JL, Fowler GC: *Procedures for primary care physicians,* St Louis, 1994, Mosby.)

Procedure

1. Obtain a history to determine the mechanism of injury, the potential for contamination, the time of occurrence, the location of the injury, tetanus immunization status, the possibility of underlying damage, and any medical history that could interfere with wound healing.

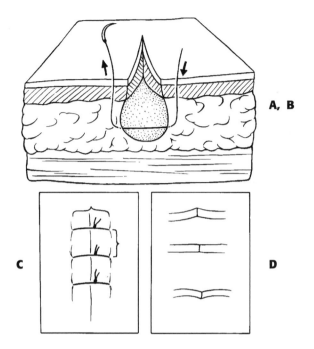

Fig. 2-5 Interrupted dermal suture. **A** Proper depth. **B** Proper spacing *(a = b)*. **C** Proper final appearance. **D** Improper final appearance. (From Pfenninger JL, Fowler GC: *Procedures for primary care physicians,* St Louis, 1994, Mosby.)

2. Examine the wound for foreign bodies, deep tissue layer damage, injury to nerve or blood vessel, or joint involvement.
3. Paint the wound's intact skin surfaces with betadine.
4. Anesthetize the wound (see Procedure on anesthesia).
5. Open the suture tray and put on sterile gloves.
6. Prepare/clean the wound. The wound can be cleaned using mechanical or chemical methods. Mechanical cleansing involves wiping, brushing, or irrigation (most important). Saline irrigation under pressure can be administered with a 30- to 60-cc syringe and an 18-gauge needle or irrigation device, using 50 to 100 cc of solution. Chemical cleaning methods include antiseptic soaps such as Shurclens and povidone–iodine scrub and are less effective.
7. Apply sterile fenestrated drapes over and around the laceration.
8. Eliminate nonviable tissue from the wound through debridement. This may be accomplished with a scalpel or sharp tissue scissors.
9. Insert sutures to approximate the wound edges. Lacerations are approximated using a variety of suturing techniques:

- A simple interrupted dermal suture (Fig. 2-5) is most commonly used. It keeps the skin margins level or slightly everted. The needle enters the skin at a right angle. The needle entrance, relative to the wound edge, is about one-half the depth of the respective dermis. The stitch should be as wide as it is deep. The distance between sutures is approximately equal to the depth of the suture, which is also equal to the distance between the suture entrance and the exit site. The knot should be tied using the instrument tie, being repeated for a total or four to five times. Do not tie the knot too tight. See Figure 2-6 on the instrument tie.
- A subcutaneous suture with an inverted knot or the "buried stitch" is used in addition to skin sutures for deep wounds or wounds under tension. Absorbable sutures are used. Begin at the bottom of the wound and come up. Go straight across

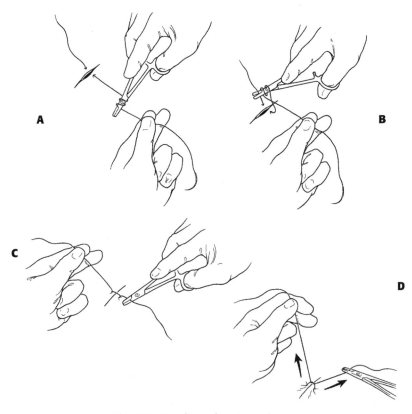

Fig. 2-6 See legend on opposite page.

the incision, then down to the base once again and tie. This places the knot most inferior in the wound (Fig. 2-7).

- The vertical mattress suture is used to produce eversion of the wound and in wounds with some tension (Fig. 2-8). See Figures 2-9 and 2-10 for the appearance of a proper wound closure.

10. Apply a nonstick dressing, then a pressure dressing if necessary for hemostasis.

Postprocedure patient education

Give the patient specific directions regarding followup care. Provide written as well as verbal instructions (see box).

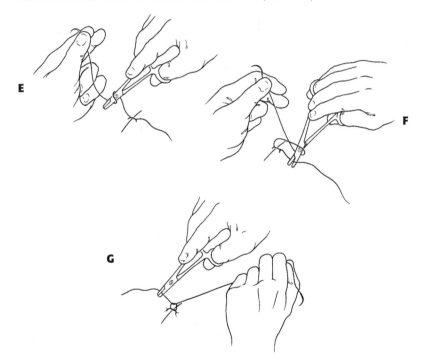

Fig. 2-6—*cont'd* Instrument tie. Manipulate the needle end of the suture with the nondominant hand and the needle holder with the dominant hand. The suture enters the far side and exits the near side of the wound. **A** Lay the needle holder on the suture on the near side and wrap the suture around the needle holder twice. **B** Reach back with the needle holder and grab the free suture end. **C** Cross hands and pull the free end back toward the near side and bring the needle end of suture to the far side. **D** Raise both suture ends and cinch the first throw. **E** Lay the needle holder on the suture on the far side and loop once. **F** Reach back and take the free suture end. **G** Cross hands to square knot. This pattern is repeated four or five times.

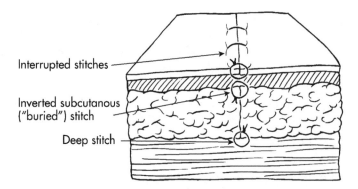

Interrupted stitches

Inverted subcutanous ("buried") stitch

Deep stitch

Fig. 2-7   Inverted subcutaneous suture. Also shown is layered closure. (From Pfenninger JL, Fowler GC: *Procedures for primary care physicians,* St Louis, 1994, Mosby.)

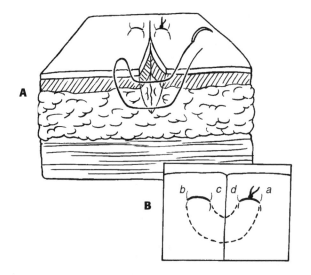

Fig. 2-8   Vertical mattress suture. **A** Cross section. **B** Overhead view. Begin at *a,* and go under skin to *b.* Come out, go in at *c,* and exit at *d.* (From Pfenninger JL, Fowler GC: *Procedures for primary care physicians,* St Louis, 1994, Mosby.)

Schedule a return visit for a wound check 2 days after suturing.

Instruct the patient to elevate the injured extremity and wear a sling when appropriate.

Direct patients to clean the wound daily with dilute hydrogen peroxide and cover with triple antibiotic ointment and a nonadhering dressing.

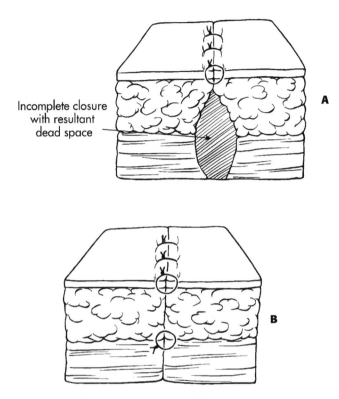

Incomplete closure
with resultant
dead space

Fig. 2-9 **A** Improper and **B** proper wound closures. (From Pfenninger JL, Fowler GC: *Procedures for primary care physicians,* St Louis, 1994, Mosby.)

Tell the patient to avoid prolonged emersion of the wound in water.

Teach the patient or the patient's parent the signs and symptoms of infection and instruct him or her to call the office if they appear (redness, increasing pain, swelling, fever, red streaks progressing up an extremity).

If the wound is over a joint, activity may need to be limited for a few days to avoid reinjuring the area or reopening the wound.

Advise patients to make liberal use of sunscreens for at least 3 to 6 months to avoid hyperpigmentation of the scar. Body image changes secondary to the presence of scars must be discussed with the patient. Warn patients that scar discoloration will be the worst at 4 to 6 weeks after the injury but will gradually fade.

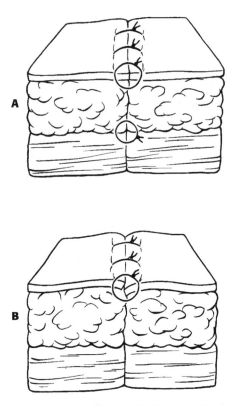

Fig. 2-10 A Proper tissue apposition and **B** inappropriate excess tightness. (From Pfenninger JL, Fowler GC: *Procedures for primary care physicians,* St Louis, 1994, Mosby.)

Practitioner Followup/Complications

If the wound shows any evidence of contamination, a 5- to 7-day course of an oral antibiotic is advisable.

Any wound with questionable viable tissue should be reexamined 24 hours after repair. Close followup will ensure early detection of infection or other wound complications.

When nonabsorbable sutures have been used, the timing of suture removal depends on the location of the wound, the thickness of the skin, and the mobility of the involved area (see box). If the wound appears to be open, leave the suture in a few more days.

COMPLICATIONS

Common complications include:

Patient Education Handout

Care of Sutured Lacerations

1. Keep wound and dressing clean. You may shower. Do not expose the wound to moisture for prolonged periods of time.
2. **Wet Dressing:** If the dressing gets wet, remove it, blot the wound dry with a sterile gauze pad, and reapply a clean, dry dressing, e.g., a sterile gauze pad.
3. **Dressing Changes:** Remove the dressing after 2 days and reapply a sterile dressing. Repeat this procedure every day until the stitches are removed, unless instructed otherwise.
4. **Signs of Infection:** If any of the following signs of infection appear, contact a physician immediately:
   a. Wound becomes red, swollen, tender, or warm.
   b. Wound begins to drain or fester.
   c. Red streaks appear around the wound.
   d. Tender lumps appear in the groin or under the arm.
   e. Chills or fever occur.
5. **Infection Check:** Because of the nature of your injury, the possibility of infection is increased. Please return to be checked in _____ days.
6. **Stitch Removal:** The physician suggests that the stitches be removed in about _____ days.
7. **Tetanus Immunization:** For your records, you/your child received the following:
   a. Tetanus Toxoid _____
   b. DT (Diphtheria-Tetanus) _____
   c. DPT (Diphtheria-Pertussis-Tetanus) _____
   d. Other _____

FROM Pfenniger JL, Fowler GC: *Procedures for primary care physicians*, St Louis, 1994, Mosby.

- Bleeding and hematoma formation
- Infection
- Skin necrosis
- Wound dehiscence
- Unfavorable features of scars
  Suture puncture marks
  Scar color

When To Remove Sutures

Area of body	Number of days
Face	3-4
Neck	4-6
Scalp	6-12
Ear	4-6
Chest or abdomen	7-12
Arm and back of hand	7-12
Legs and top of feet	10-14
Back	7-12
Palms and soles	7-14

To remove suture

1. Clean the area with Betadine.
2. Cut suture at skin entry on the side opposite the knot.
3. With clamps or pickups, pull on the knot.
4. Suture should be easily removed.
5. If sutures are crusted over, wash the area with Betadine or warm water to remove crusts before removing the sutures.
6. Determine whether the wound needs further care (steri-strips or dressing changes). If wound healing is compromised because of steroid use or systemic disease such as diabetes, sutures can remain in place for 2 or 3 weeks.

Scar depression or elevation
Hypertrophic scarring and keloids

CPT BILLING CODES

12001—Simple repair is used when the wound is superficial (e.g., involving primarily epidermis or dermis, or subcutaneous tissues without significant involvement of deeper structures) and requires simple one-layer closure/suturing. This includes local anesthesia and chemical or electrocauterization of wounds not closed.

12031—Intermediate repair includes the repair of wounds that, in addition to the above, require layered closure of one or more of the deeper layers of subcutaneous tissue and superficial (nonmuscle) fascia, in addition to the skin (epidermal and dermal) closure. Single-layer closure of heavily contaminated wounds that have required extensive cleaning or removal of particulate matter also constitutes intermediate repair.

BIBLIOGRAPHY

Boriskin MI: Primary care management of wounds, *Nurse Practitioner* 19(11):38, 1994.
Byrne JJ: Hand infections—the academic surgeon's perspective, *Postgrad Med* 80(7):112, 1986.
Codner M, Jones G: Repair techniques for facial wounds, *Emerg Med* 26(2):26, 1994.
Kravis TC, Warner CG, Jacobs LM: *Emergency medicine: a comprehensive review,* New York, 1993, Raven Press.
Rosen J: Emergency wound management, *Top Emerg Med* 11(1): 1989.
Rosen P, Barkin RM, Sternbach GL: *Essentials of Emergency Medicine,* Baltimore, 1991, Mosby.
Rosen R, and others: *Emergency medicine. Concepts and clinical practice,* St Louis, 1988, Mosby.
Schmitt BD: *Instructions for pediatric patients,* Philadelphia, 1992, WB Saunders.

Elliptical Excision and Biopsy

Description

This is a common procedure used to remove a suspicious or miscellaneous skin lesion. Because sufficient tissue must be obtained for an accurate diagnosis, the entire lesion with full dermal thickness sampling is removed for biopsy. Biopsy is indicated with all skin lesions that are suspected of being neoplasms.

Indications

Excision and biopsy are used for the following reasons.

- To make or confirm a diagnosis for definitive treatment
- To excise and thus cure the lesion
- To perform elective removal for cosmetic reasons

Contraindications/Precautions

Practitioners should not attempt the procedure if there is an infection at the site of the proposed biopsy.

Practitioners should not perform the procedure if the patient has a bleeding disorder (or coagulopathy) of sufficient consequence that hemostasis would be difficult.

The practitioner should not perform the procedure if the patient has an allergy to local anesthetics.

Deep lesions or lesions on the face should be referred to a dermatologist or plastic surgeon.

Patient Preparation/Education

While draping and positioning the patient, practitioners should reassure and relax the patient. Remind the patient that this is a sterile procedure and the patient will need to keep hands out of the area. Discuss how pain will be controlled.

Equipment

- Fine scissors to cut hair
- Sterile gloves
- Sterile field
- Sterile drape
- Betadine
- Injectable lidocaine 1% and syringe
- Sterile 4 × 4 gauze
- Sterile normal saline
- Dissecting forceps
- Scalpel with blade (size No. 10, 11, or 15)
- Sharp curettage
- Needle holders
- Suture material
- Skin hooks
- Antibacterial ointment

Procedure

1. Position the patient so that the lesion is easily accessible.
2. Adhere to sterile technique throughout the procedure.
3. Clean the area on and around the lesion with Betadine.
4. Cut, do not shave, any hair around the lesion.

5. Place sterile drape(s) around the lesion.
6. Anesthetize: Inject lidocaine with or without epinephrine (depending on the site—see anesthesia protocol) into the subcutaneous skin around the area involved. Allow a few minutes for the medication to take effect.
7. Make an elliptical incision around the lesion. The ellipse should be three times as long as it is wide and should lie parallel to the skin tension lines (Fig. 2-11).
8. Excise the tissue within the incision to include the lesion and the necessary margin of normal skin (Fig. 2-12).
9. With the dissecting forceps, pull the lesion and its contents out *en bloc.*
10. Use a sharp curettage to remove any remaining lesion wall.
11. Close the skin opening. See suturing procedure for details. The suturing technique used should be simple interrupted for most excisions because it permits good eversion of the wound edges. Use a layered suturing technique if the areais deep. This helps to relieve the tension of skin closure, evert skin edges, and

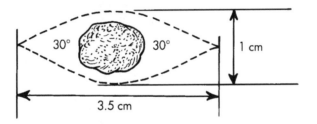

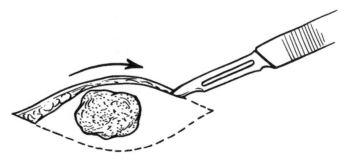

Fig. 2-11 Elliptical excision biopsy technique. (From Pfenninger JL, Fowler GC: *Procedures for primary care physicians,* St Louis, 1994, Mosby.)

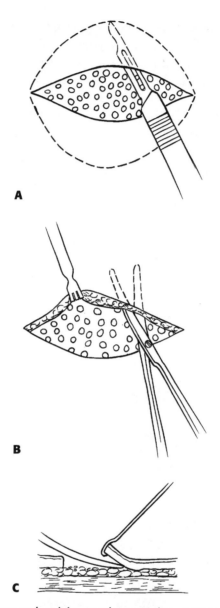

Fig. 2-12 Subcutaneous undermining to release tension on wound margins. **A** with scalpel and **B** with scissors. This also aids eversion of edges during closure. **C** Proper level for undermining within subcutaneous fat. (From Pfenninger JL, Fowler GC: *Procedures for primary care physicians,* St Louis, 1994, Mosby.)

minimize dead space and hematoma formations. Use an absorbable suture material such as chromic gut for closure in layers. If the lesion is in hairbearing scalp, close the wound with absorbable suture. This will leave stitch mark scars, but they will be hidden by hair, and the patient need not return for suture removal.

12. Should dog ears appear at the ends of the wound, remove them as follows: Insert a skin hook in the end of the incision and elevate the excess tissue. On one side of this tissue, make an incision at its base, pull the resulting skin flap across the wound, and remove the excess skin. Finally, suture the remaining section of the incision.

13. Using a sterile 4 × 4 gauze, clean the sutured wound of any blood with normal saline.

14. Apply a thin layer of antibacterial ointment to the incision and cover it with a sterile gauze.

15. Instruct the patient in proper wound care (see Postprocedure patient education).

16. Remove sutures in 7 to 10 days. If necessary, apply steri-strips at that time to reinforce wound.

Postprocedure patient education

Instruct the patient to keep the wound clean and dry.

Review signs and symptoms of infection with the patient. These include redness, increasing pain, swelling, fever, or red streaks progressing up an extremity.

Instruct the patient to return to the office should these symptoms develop.

Instruct the patient to return to the office in 7 to 10 days for suture removal.

Practitioner Followup/Complications

Infection of the wound after surgical closure can be managed with incision and drainage, placement of iodoform gauze into the wound, and appropriate antibiotics.

Follow up with the patient regarding the results of biopsy and inform him or her if any further treatment is necessary.

CPT BILLING CODES

Excision is defined as full-thickness (through the dermis) removal of lesions and simple closure and includes local anesthesia.

11400-11406—Excision, benign lesion, except skin tag, trunk, arms, or legs.

11420-11426—Excision benign lesion, except skin tag, scalp, neck, hands, feet, genitalia.

11440-11446—Excision, other benign lesion, face, ears, eyelids, nose, lips, mucous membrane.

BIBLIOGRAPHY

Hughes N: *Basic techniques of excision and wound closure.* In Barclay T, Kernahan D, editors: *Rob & Smith's operative surgery: plastic surgery,* ed 4, Boston, 1991, Butterworths.

Pfenninger JL, Fowler GC: *Procedures for primary care physicians,* St Louis, 1994, Mosby.

Reeves J, Maibach H: *Clinical dermatology illustrated: a regional approach,* ed 2, Philadelphia, 1991, F.A. Davis.

Roberts PW: *Useful procedures in medical practice,* Philadelphia, 1986, Lea & Febiger.

Abscess Incision and Drainage

Description

A cutaneous abscess is a localized collection of pus resulting in a painful, fluctuant, soft tissue mass surrounded by firm granulation tissue and erythema.

Indications

Incision and drainage (I&D) is done to reduce pressure and tissue damage to surrounding tissues. It is indicated only when the skin is tense because of a localized collection of pus, with surrounding firm granulation tissue and erythema. A small abscess or one that is not tense should be treated with warm compresses until it either resolves spontaneously or becomes tense. Culture and sensitivity testing of abscess material should be considered.

Contraindications/Precautions

Practitioners do not perform I&D if it is not possible to achieve adequate anesthesia.

The procedure is contraindicated in the presence of a deep foreign body.

The patient should be referred to a specialist if the abscess is in proximity to vascular, nervous, or tendinous structures.

The patient should be referred to a specialist if there is hand, joint, perirectal, periurethral, or facial involvement.

Patients with signs or symptoms of systemic involvement, or patients who are diabetic or immunosuppressed, should be referred because they may need hospitalization for incision and drainage.

Patient Preparation/Education

The practitioner gives the rationale for incision and drainage (and culture and sensitivity if indicated).

The patient should be assured that pain will decrease after the pressure is relieved and pus is drained.

Equipment

- Betadine
- Scissors if necessary to remove hair
- Sterile drape
- Sterile gloves
- Lidocaine 1% and 5-cc syringe with 25-gauge needle, or ethyl chloride spray
- 10-cc syringe with 22-gauge needle for aspiration (optional)
- Scalpel with No. 11 blade
- Culture swab (optional)
- Hydrogen peroxide
- Sterile cotton-tip swab
- Normal saline
- Forceps
- Irrigating syringe with 18-gauge angiocath and basin
- ¼ or ½ inch plain strip gauze (or iodoform strip gauze)

- Sterile scissors
- 4 × 4 gauze pads
- Tape

Procedure

1. Position the patient and the site to allow for good site visibility and the patient's comfort.
2. Gently scrub the site and surrounding the area with Betadine for 1 to 2 minutes, removing excess hair if necessary for visualization.
3. Drape.
4. Administer anesthesia. (See also Procedure on anesthesia.) Anesthesia is not necessary for I&D of a paronychia in a child.
   Ethyl Chloride spray: used for superficial lesions with obvious fluctuance. Prepare the patient for the cooling effect by demonstrating on your own hand, then the patient's hand; then spray the lesion, maintaining steady spray until frost appears—proceed to step 5 immediately.
   Lidocaine 1%: used for deep lesions or those too large for single brief incision. Infiltrate intradermally along proposed incision line, limiting injection sites and using the minimal solution necessary for effective anesthesia to minimize induration; may use ring-block infiltration of lidocaine approximately 1 cm from erythematous peripheral border of abscess.
5. Locate fluctuance by a two-finger gentle pressure; resort to fine-needle aspiration if fluctuance is questionable (not when fluctuance is absent), using the 22-gauge needle to demonstrate pus.

Important: Do not proceed with the incision if fluctuance or purulence cannot be demonstrated! (Prescribe moist heat and elevation for 24 hours, treat any existing cellulitis, and reexamine.)

6. With demonstrated fluctuance, and when anesthesia is achieved, make a single quick incision parallel to the natural skin lines from edge to edge across the fluctuance where pus has been demonstrated by fine-needle aspiration, or make a single stab incision following the needle path (Fig. 2-13). Ex-

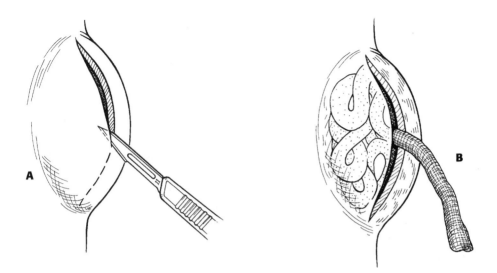

Fig. 2-13 Incision and drainage of an abscess. Prepare and drape the area. Inject 1% to 2% lidocaine around the perimeter of the abscess, taking care not to infiltrate the abscess cavity. **A** Make an incision sufficiently wide to allow drainage and prevent premature closure, which could result in recollection of pus and recurrence of the abscess. **B** Place a drain. In this case, iodoform gauze is used. (From Pfenninger JL, Fowler GC: *Procedures for primary care physicians,* St Louis, 1994, Mosby.)

pect spontaneous drainage of some pus, which may be mixed with blood. If no spontaneous flow occurs, try light pressure over the surrounding skin (do not apply pressure if the lesion is on the patient's face or mastoid).

7. Collect a culture specimen, if indicated.
8. Probe the abscess with a hydrogen peroxide–soaked cotton-tip swab to break up debris. Remember that abscesses are usually irregular in shape, with fingerlike projections.
9. Irrigate the site thoroughly with normal saline, using the lidocaine syringe and the angiocath needle, until pus is no longer obtained. Observe for bleeding.
10. Packing will stop slight oozing, but in the unusual case of persistent bleeding use silver nitrate sticks to cauterize.
11. Hold the incision open and use forceps to pack the wound with ¼ or ½ inch strip gauze (plain or iodoform). Fill the cavity tightly enough to cause hemostasis but not so tightly that it causes pain.
12. Cover the wound with 4 × 4 gauze and secure with tape.

Postprocedure patient education

Inform the patient to expect some oozing (pus, exudate, scant bleeding).

Demonstrate how to cover the wound with gauze.

Instruct the patient to use warm peroxide and water (in a ratio of 1:1) soaks 2 to 4 times a day for 1 week, followed by redressing.

Instruct the patient not to attempt repacking the wound if the packing falls out.

Reemphasize that healing takes 1 to 3 weeks, depending on the size, depth, and location of the wound.

Notify practitioner if drainage increases, healing is problematic, or fever develops.

Practitioner Followup/Complications

Practitioners may be called upon to reevaluate a facial wound treated by a specialists 24 hours after the incision and drainage.

The site should be checked every 1 to 3 days depending on the size of the lesion, resolution of erythema and drainage, and patient reliability.

Practitioners remove the packing and assess the patient's response to treatment. If a large amount of drainage persists, repack the cavity.

When erythema is resolving and drainage is minimal, discontinue the packing.

After the packing is removed the patient should be instructed to use warm soaks 3 to 4 times a day for 10 to 15 minutes over 2 to 3 days.

Healing should occur in 5 to 9 days.

Bleeding may occur in highly vascular areas, or in conditions of excessive pressure or trauma to the granulation tissue. Pack the site, provide pressure to the source, or cauterize.

Recurrence of the abscess is a result of inadequate incision, incomplete probing, inadequate irrigation, or poor postcare. Reincise the old incision site, and drain and irrigate aggressively.

CPT BILLING CODES

10060—Incision and drainage of abscess (e.g., carbuncle, suppurative hidradenitis, cutaneous or subcutaneous abscess, cyst, furuncle, or paronychia; simple or single.

10061—Complicated or multiple.

10140—Incision and drainage of hematoma, seroma, or fluid collection.

BIBLIOGRAPHY

Caruthers LD, Griggs R, Snell GF: Office management of epithelial cysts and cutaneous abscesses, *Primary Care* 13(3):477, 1986.

Ghurch J: The treatment of infections and abscesses, *Practitioner* 232(1444):255, 1988.

Graber RF: Procedures for your practice: incision and drainage of cutaneous abscesses, *Patient Care* 20(2):163, 1986.

Ho M: *Current emergency diagnosis and treatment,* ed 3, Norwalk, Conn, 1990, Appleton & Lange.

Rosen P, Barkin R, Braen R: *Emergency medicine: concepts and clinical practice,* ed 3, St Louis, 1992, Mosby.

Cyst Removal

Description

This protocol describes the technique commonly used to remove a cyst. A cyst is an enclosed sac of dermis or subcutaneous layers under the skin, lined with epithelium and containing fluid or semisolid material. The epidermal cyst, or sebaceous cyst, is a round, tense, keratinizing cyst that is freely mobile and very superficial. There may or may not be a history of drainage or inflammation with purulent discharge. Cysts are most often found on the face, scalp, neck, and back and range in size from a few millimeters to 5 cm. Examination reveals a fairly firm, smooth, flesh-colored, freely movable nodule with a small central pore.

Indications

Removal may be for cosmetic reasons or to prevent recurrent episodes of infection.

Contraindications/Precautions

Practitioners do not attempt cyst removal if a deep foreign body is present.

Practitioners do not operate if there is inflammation of the cyst (perform I&D—see I&D procedure).

Practitioners should proceed carefully if the cyst is in close proximity to vascular, nervous, or tendinous structures.

Practitioners should not attempt removal if the cyst has hand or joint involvement.

Practitioners should not attempt with perirectal, periurethral, or facial involvement.

Practitioners should avoid cyst incision in patients with signs or symptoms of systemic involvement, or patients who are diabetic or immunosuppressed.

Patient Preparation/Education

Practitioners assure the patient that pain will decrease after the pressure is relieved and pus is drained.

Practitioners warn the patient to expect a tugging sensation.

Equipment

- Sterile gloves
- Betadine
- Topical or local anesthesia (See Anesthesia procedure)
- Scalpel with a No. 11 blade
- Curved hemostats
- Culture swab (optional)
- Normal saline
- Irrigating syringe with 18-gauge angiocath and basin
- ¼ or ½ inch plain strip gauze (or iodoform strip gauze)
- Sterile scissors
- 4 × 4 gauze pads
- Tape

Procedure

1. Clean the cyst and its margins with Betadine.
2. Use topical anesthesia for a small cyst or local anesthesia for deep cysts and those too large for a single, brief incision (see Anesthesia procedure).
3. With the scalpel, make a small incision into the cyst.
4. Express the contents of the cyst by applying light pressure at the cyst margins.
5. Frequently, this external pressure extrudes not only the sebaceous material of the cyst, but the sac itself. If the sac is not pulled loose, then insert curved hemostats into the wound and make repeated attempts to grasp the sac and pull it out in its entirety.
6. Collect a culture specimen, if indicated.
7. Irrigate the site thoroughly with normal saline, using a syringe and an angiocath needle.
8. Pack the wound with ¼ or ½ inch strip gauze. Fill the cavity tightly enough to cause hemostasis but not so tightly that it causes pain.
9. Cover the wound with 4 × 4 gauze and secure with tape.

Postprocedure patient education

Inform the patient to expect some oozing (pus, exudate, scant bleeding).

Instruct the patient not to attempt repacking of the wound if the packing falls out.

Instruct the patient to notify the practitioner if any of the signs and symptoms of infection occur: redness, increasing pain, swelling, fever, or red streaks progressing up an extremity.

Inform the patient that healing occurs from the inside out as the iodoform gauze is gradually removed. This will entail several visits to the practitioner's office for close followup.

After removing the packing, instruct the patient to use warm soaks 3 to 4 times a day for 10 to 15 minutes over 2 to 3 days.

Practitioner Followup/Complications

The practitioner should have the patient return to the office in 1 to 2 days and then every 2 to 3 days after that for gradual removal of packing and assessment of wound healing.

When erythema is resolving and drainage is minimal, the packing can be discontinued. If a large amount of drainage persists, the cavity may have to be repacked.

Recurrence of the cyst may be caused by sac adherence or incomplete removal of the sac. Full excisional removal of cyst by a surgeon is then recommended.

CPT BILLING CODES

10060—Incision and drainage of abscess (e.g., carbuncle, suppurative hidradenitis, cutaneous or subcutaneous abscess, cyst, furuncle, or paronychia); simple or single.

10061—Complicated or multiple.

BIBLIOGRAPHY

Caruthers LD, Griggs R, Snell GF: Office management of epithelial cysts and cutaneous abscesses, *Primary Care* 13(3):477, 1986.

Klin B, Ashkenazi H: Sebaceous cyst excision with minimal surgery, *Am Fam Physician* 41(6):1746, 1990.

Pfenninger JL, Fowler GC: *Procedures for primary care physicians,* St Louis, 1994, Mosby.

Skin Tag Removal–Cautery or Snipping

Description

Practitioners are often asked to surgically remove a skin tag (or acrochordon), which is a pedunculated papilloma occurring on the eyelids, neck, axillae, or groin. If the skin tag is large enough, elliptical excision can be used as described under that procedure. This procedure describes cauterization and removal by snipping.

Skin tags occur more in females and obese individuals. They are usually asymptomatic, although they can become tender and inflamed after twisting of the stalk or trauma to the area. On examination, skin tags are flesh colored to hyperpigmented, vary in size from less than 1 mm to more than 10 mm, are round to oval, and are soft and pliable. They should be differentiated from pedunculated seborrheic keratosis, dermal or compound melanocytic nevus, neurofibroma, or molluscum contagiosum.

Indications

Skin tags are removed for cosmetic reasons.

Contraindications/Precautions

Snipping should not be attempted if there is a history of hypertrophic scarring or keloid formation after surgery.

Practitioners may choose to refer patients with skin tags on the eyelids to a dermatologist.

Practitioners should refer all skin tags on the face of a child to a dermatologist.

Patient Preparation/Education

Practitioners inform the patient that local anesthesia is usually not required for tags less than 1 cm. The patient may feel a slight burning sensation with liquid nitrogen or a tugging sensation if tags are removed with scissors.

The patient should be advised that a small depression can form at the site of the tag when it is removed from the face.

The practitioner reviews the procedure with the patient to include use of a local anesthetic agent if needed, removal of skin tags by electrocautery, or scissors.

The patient should be advised to remain still during the procedure and to notify the practitioner of any discomfort.

The practitioner reviews risks associated with the procedure, including bleeding, infection, and scarring, with the patient.

Equipment

Electrocautery
- Anesthesia optional—see Anesthesia chapter

- Cautery tool (electric) with a fine tip

Snipping
- Forceps
- Sterile scissors
- Silver nitrate sticks or solution or other styptic
- Sterile dressing (optional)

Procedure

Tags removed with electrocautery
1. Anesthesia is not required for tags less than 1 cm.
2. Larger tags will require local topical anesthesia and electro-cautery to control bleeding.
3. Use a fine-tipped electric cautery tool with a cool setting and apply cautery lightly to the skin tag.

Tags removed by snipping with scissors
1. Small tags can be snipped without anesthesia.
2. Grasp the fold of skin between thumb and index finger to position tag on its apex. This allows tag to be snipped without inadvertently cutting or pinching surrounding skin.
3. Quickly snip the tag.
4. Apply silver nitrate stick or other styptic to area to stop bleeding.

Postprocedure patient education
Inform the patient that tags will appear red and be tender after cauterization and will dry up and fall off.

Advise the patient that tags removed by scissors may bleed after the procedure. The patient may need to apply pressure with a dressing.

Instruct the patient to keep areas clean and dry.

Review signs and symptoms of infection with the patient. Give instruction to return to the clinic if any redness, pain, swelling, or fever develops.

Practitioner Followup/Complications

No followup is necessary unless complications occur.
The most common complication is infection.

CPT/BILLING CODES

The procedure is defined as removal by scissoring, or any sharp method or ligature strangulation, including chemical or electrocauterization of wound, with or without local anesthesia.

11200—Removal of skin tags, multiple fibrocutaneous tags, any area; up to and including 15 lesions.

11201—Each additional ten lesions.

BIBLIOGRAPHY

Madden S: *Current dermatological therapy,* Philadelphia, 1991, WB Saunders.
Pfenninger JL, Fowler GC: *Procedures for primary care physicians,* St Louis, 1994, Mosby.
Reeves J, Maibach H: *Clinical dermatology illustrated: a regional approach,* ed 2, Philadelphia, 1991, FA Davis.

Wart Removal—Chemical and Cryotherapy

Description

Warts (verrucae) are common, benign epithelial tumors, viral in origin, that occur on the skin or mucous membrane. All warts are mildly contagious and have an incubation period (after inoculation) of one to several months, the average time being 2 to 18 months.

Common warts (verrucae vulgaris) are almost universal in the population, and most do not become malignant. They are sharply demarcated, rough surfaced, round or irregular, firm, light gray, yellow, brown, or grayish-black tumors 2 to 10 mm in diameter. They appear most frequently on sites subject to trauma (e.g., fingers, elbows, knees, face, scalp) but may spread elsewhere.

Periungual warts are common warts occurring around the nail plate. Plantar warts (verrucae plantaris) are common warts on the sole of the foot; they are flattened by pressure and surrounded by cornified epithelium. They may be exquisitely tender and can be distinguished from corns and calluses by their tendency to pinpoint bleeding when the surface is pared away. Mosaic warts are plaques of myriad small, closely set plantar warts.

Filiform warts are long, narrow, small growths usually seen on the eyelids, face, neck, or lips. Flat warts are smooth, flat, yellow-brown lesions and occur more commonly in children and young adults, most often on the face and along scratch marks through autoinoculation. Warts of unusual shape—e.g., pedunculated or resembling a cauliflower—are most frequent on the head and neck, especially on the scalp and bearded region.

As with most viral infections, warts occur more commonly in children, and they go away when immunity develops. In young children, warts may last just a few months, in older children they may last about a year, and in adults they may last for months to years. Most warts go away spontaneously and heal without scars.

Warts may behave differently in different locations. Warts around the fingernails and on the palms and soles are particularly long lived and stubborn. Warts on the beard area of men who shave are particularly troublesome because shaving often spreads them, as does shaving of legs in women. In the same way, picking at or chewing of warts on the hands may spread them, especially under the fingernails. Warts caused by the human papilloma virus may grow profusely on the geni-

---

Types of Treatments Available for Common Warts

1. Chemical destruction

     Salicylic acid solutions
     Cantharadine
     Podophyllin

2. Cryotherapy using liquid nitrogen
3. Curettage with electrodesiccation—Refer to a physician
4. Surgical or laser excision—Refer to a physician
5. Intralesional injection (bleomycin)—Refer to a physician
6. Immunotherapy—Usually refer to a physician

talia of adults and can be passed between sexual partners. See the box for available treatments. Procedures to be discussed in this text will be wart removal by chemical destruction and by cryotherapy.

Indications

All treatments work by tissue destruction, the goal being to destroy the virus-containing epidermis and preserve as much uninvolved tissue as possible. The type and aggressiveness of therapy will depend on the type of wart, its location, and the patient's cooperation and immune status. The least painful methods should be used initially, especially in young children. More destructive therapies should be reserved for areas where scarring is not a consideration or for recalcitrant lesions.

A major point to remember when treating warts is that the virus is microscopic, and although after treatment the skin may look normal, there often is virus still present in remaining tissue. Unless that tissue also is removed, a few months later the warts will recur. Therefore all treatments should attempt to remove several layers of skin beyond the first signs of normal tissue. Such therapy may take several weeks or even months, but patience and perseverance are essential. Patients should never be guaranteed that the initial removal of a wart will be the definitive treatment.

Plantar warts should be treated with nonscarring methods if at all possible, because a scar on the sole of the foot can be quite painful and is irreversible. Therefore, only severe, recalcitrant plantar lesions should be considered for possible treatment with curettage and desiccation or excision.

Periungual warts usually require no treatment if they are not painful. Patients should be instructed to stop nail and cuticle biting. Warts on the proximal nail fold must be treated gently to avoid permanent injury to the underlying nail bed; this would result in permanent nail deformity.

Contraindications/Precautions

A history of adverse reaction to the treatment methods contraindicates the procedure.

Caution must be used when removing warts from patients with diabetes or who are immunocompromised.

Chemical treatments are contraindicated in pregnant women.

Usually no more than five warts are removed at any one time.

Chemical Destruction

Patient Preparation/Education

Chemical treatment of warts causes the epithelium to swell, soften, macerate, and then desquamate. Treatment may become progressively more painful as wart tissue macerates and the chemical reaches more sensitive epidermal and dermal tissue.

The practitioner should inform patients about the high rate of recurrence; they may need multiple treatments.

Equipment

SALICYLIC ACID PROCEDURE
- White bandage tape (not paper tape)
- Adhesive bandage with center cut out to fit around wart.
- Salicylic acid preparation. Salicylic acid preparations come in various strengths. Stronger preparations usually are reserved for thicker areas (e.g., palms, soles, extremities), and weaker strengths for the digits of younger children. Duofilm, Salactol, compound W (salicylic acid 6.7% and lactic acid 16.7%), or occlusal HP (salicylic acid 17%) allows easy application on multiple sites and is useful for common plantar and palmar warts. Duoplant (salicylic acid 27%) is a stronger concentration useful for thicker lesions. Mediplast (salicylic acid 40%) is especially useful for plantar warts and is best applied to the wart and a few millimeters of surrounding normal skin. Keralyt, Cuplex (salicylic acid 6 to 11%) or salicylic acid 20 to 40% plaster (self-adhesive corn plaster) can be used on plantar warts.

CANTHARIDIN 0.7% PROCEDURE
- Cantharidin 0.7%

- Clear tape
- Triple antibiotic ointment

15% PODOPHYLLIN PAINT PROCEDURE
- Vinegar
- Cotton tipped applicators
- Podophyllin paint 15%

Procedure

Procedure for salicylic acid

This procedure can be taught so that the patient can perform it at home.

1. Soak the affected area in warm water for 5 to 10 minutes.
2. Put a bandage with the center cut out around the wart to prevent maceration of surrounding skin.
3. Cover the wart with the chemical solution and allow it to dry. The compound turns white when it is dry. Blowing on it or using a fan makes it dry faster. Apply at bedtime.
4. Cover with white bandage tape to seal out the air. This macerates the wart skin and cause the acid solution to penetrate much better. Do not use paper tape or tape with holes in it that breathes. It is not harmful to get the tape wet as long as it stays in place.
5. Remove the tape after 48 to 72 hours. Peel off as much of the wart skin as possible. A small knife, emery board, or razor blade may be used to remove any remaining wart tissue.
6. Do not retreat the wart for 24 hours or the medicine may sting and irritate the affected area. The wart is much more tender just after peeling.
7. Repeat the process until all of the wart is removed and only pink skin is left on the affected area.
8. When the wart appears to be gone, check at least weekly for any early recurrence. The earlier a recurrence is seen and treatment is initiated, the easier it will be to clear the wart permanently.
9. To obtain maximum benefit, it may be necessary to continue treatment for as long as 3 months. Contamination of the sur-

rounding skin causes irritation, and there is often discomfort before the wart is cured.

Procedure for cantharidin 0.7%

Cantharidin is an extract of the blister beetle and may be useful in conjunction with salicylic acid preparations or between treatments. If the patient is very responsive, he or she may only need one treatment, followed by application of a salicylic acid preparation.

1. Apply cantharidin carefully to the individual lesions following the same guidelines used for salicylic acid.
2. Cover with clear tape.
3. Blistering will occur within 2 to 24 hours, after which time the tape should be removed and the medication washed off with soap and water.
4. Use triple antibiotic ointment to exposed areas twice daily.
5. Blistering may be very uncomfortable, and the chemotoxic response varies among patients; some have swelling with pain, others have no response at all. The application itself is painless.

Procedure for 15% Podophyllin paint

Use on moist areas such as the glans of the uncircumcised penis, the vagina and vulva, the perineal area, and the groin. Use for small warts. Identify warts by brushing vinegar over the area. The infected area shows up as a white patch.

Avoid using podophyllin if genital warts are extensive because toxicity may result from systemic absorption. If overused, podophyllin may result in polyneuritis, ileus, paresthesias, fever, leukopenia, and thrombopenia.

1. A cotton-tipped applicator is dipped in the solution and wrung out by rolling it inside the neck of the bottle.
2. Carefully single out individual warts and touch them with the solution.

Postprocedure patient education

Instruct the patients to wash Podophyllin off 4 to 6 hours after treatment. Ibuprofen is suggested for pain relief from blisters.

Screen patients for other sexually transmitted disease along with examination of their sexual partners.

Patients may require analgesics for pain.

Advise the patients that if irritation or soreness occurs, the treatment should be temporarily stopped and then resumed several days later.

Tell the patients to check for reoccurrence weekly and treat immediately if the wart reappears.

Educate patients about how warts are spread and encourage them to use condoms.

Practitioner Followup/Complications

Warts may recur.

Several treatments of warts may be necessary.

Treated warts should be monitored for signs of infection.

Cryotherapy

Cryotherapy uses cold as a destructive medium. Cryogenic materials include carbon dioxide ($-78.5°$ C), liquid nitrous oxide ($-89.5°$ C) and liquid nitrogen ($-195.6°$ C). Liquid nitrogen is considered to be the most useful because of its low temperature, easy availability, low cost, and safety. Liquid nitrogen evaporates very quickly once exposed to room air, so it is stored in metal Dewar containers.

Liquid nitrogen is effective for warts on the face, around the eyes, nose, and mouth, including the mucosa. It is safe to use in children and in pregnant women. However, the treatment may be too painful in small children with multiple warts.

Common warts (verrucae vulgaris) and plantar warts (verrucae plantaris) are usually treated with cotton swabs. Mosaic warts, flat warts, and condylomata acuminata are usually spray frozen.

Cryotherapy is especially useful for warts that have failed to respond to 3 months of topical treatment and for facial warts. Cryotherapy is rarely successful with just one treatment because of the depth of the wart; however, repeated treatments may be successful.

Patient Preparation/Education

During the treatment, the patient may feel no pain or, at the most, a burning sensation.

Moderate to severe throbbing pain occurs after the treatment and usually lasts from several minutes to many hours, depending on the location and size of the affected area.

If hyperkeratosis is present, 10% salicylic ointment should be applied to the wart for several days before treatment.

Equipment

- Liquid nitrogen, in either a styrofoam container or a metal Dewar container with a spray applicator.
- Sterile cotton-tipped applicators, if nitrogen is in a styrofoam container. The diameter of the cotton tip applicator should be more or less the same as the diameter of the lesion. Standard cotton swabs usually need to be loosened or have additional cotton rolled onto the swab for a better matrix to hold the liquid.

Procedure

1. Dip the prepared cotton tip in the liquid nitrogen.
2. Press the tip firmly against the lesion. Hold the applicator in perpendicularly against the lesion until a white frozen halo (the "ice ball") appears that extends 2 to 3 mm beyond the base of the lesion. Pressure on the swab increases the depth of the penetration.
3. The time of freezing varies, depending on the type of wart and its depth, diameter, and location. It may vary from a few seconds (15 to 30 seconds) for verrucae plana to about 90 seconds for verrucae plantaris.
4. Directly after the treatment, the treated area first becomes pale and then turns red. After a few minutes, a swelling occurs, which may last several hours. Later, serous or blood-filled blisters will form. The blister should cover the whole lesion with a several millimeter margin around it; however, it should not extend significantly beyond the frozen area.

5. Do not remove the roof of the blister because this may lead to infection of the uncovered area. The blister covering serves as protection from organisms and eliminates the need for a bandage.
6. After a few days, the blister dries up, and a scab forms that lasts 1 or 2 weeks. The lesion is usually healed within 3 weeks.
7. Recommend a followup visit to determine whether viable wart tissue remains at the base of the healed blister. If remaining wart tissue is found, followup treatment is needed.
8. For the spray method, use changeable nozzles adapted to the shape and diameter of the lesions. The nozzle should be held close to the skin to prevent spraying the surrounding areas. Freeze plane warts by the spray method for a few seconds (very superficially), enough to bring an inflammatory reaction but not to produce blisters. Mosaic warts should be frozen superficially but sufficiently to produce blisters (15 to 30 seconds). For condylomata acuminata, the period of freezing lasts from a few seconds for small lesions to between 20 and 30 seconds for large ones. Avoid spraying numerous lesions during a single procedure because this leads to swelling. Condylomata acuminata disappear more rapidly than ordinary warts. Therefore, reexamine the patient after 7 to 14 days.

Practitioner Followup/Complication

Infection of the lesion should be watched for after treatment. Practitioners should check for recurrence of lesion.

There are some reports in the literature of fever lasting for 2 to 3 days, hypertrophic scars in patients with tendency to keloids, and neuropathy caused by treatment that is reversible within a period of several weeks to months.

Practitioners may consider referring patients when warts do not respond to treatment, when they are excessively numerous, or when they are on the face or in areas that may disfigure from scarring.

If warts do not respond to conventional treatment as outlined in this procedure within three treatment interventions, then a referral to a dermatologist may be indicated.

Spontaneous regression may occur in as many as two thirds of warts within 2 years. However, new warts may appear while others are regressing.

CPT BILLING CODES

17110—Destruction by any method of flat (plane, juvenile) warts or molluscum contagiosum, milia, up to 15 lesions. (Retreatment same as office visit.)

BIBLIOGRAPHY

Beutner KR: Bridging the gap. Notes of a wart watcher, *Arch Dermatol* 126(11):1432, 1990.
Bolton RA: Nongenital warts: classification and treatment options, *Am Fam Physician* 43(6):2049, 1991.
Dachow-Siwiec E: Technique of cryotherapy, *Clin Dermatol* 3(4):185, 1985.
Taylor MB: Successful treatment of warts. Choosing the best method for each situation, *Postgrad Med* 84(8):126, 1988.

Ulcer Debridement

Description

Debridement is the removal of foreign materials and necrotic or contaminated tissue from or adjacent to a traumatic or infected lesion until the surrounding healthy tissue is exposed. The devitalized tissue must be removed because it serves as a growth medium for bacteria. Healthy granulation tissue will not grow in the presence of large numbers of bacteria, and epithelial cells will not grow across surfaces contaminated by dead or foreign material.

There are two techniques for the removal of necrotic material: surgical excision and topical debriding agents.

Surgical excision is considered to be the most effective method of debridement. It involves the excision of devitalized tissue surrounding the wound. The resulting wound bed is left clean and bleeding, and the wound can then granulate freely.

If surgical excision is not indicated, topical debriding agents may be considered. A variety of chemical agents, enzyme preparations, and hygroscopic agents may be used as an alternative to the more aggressive approach of surgical excision. Chemical agents break down tissue and have an antibacterial action on the surface of the necrotic material. Enzyme preparations contain proteolytic enzymes. Hygroscopic agents act by hydrophilic action, which draws the fluid from the wound bed and absorbs the moist exudate and liquid debris.

Contraindications/Precautions

Refer the wound if:

- Its size is greater than 10 cm
- Its depth is greater than 1 cm
- It is painful
- It is a wound of the face, hand, or forearm
- Infection is present

Patient Preparation/Education

The procedure should not be painful.

Equipment

SURGICAL EXCISION
- Sterile gloves
- Sterile forceps
- Scissors or scalpel, 15 gauge
- Gauze

TOPICAL DEBRIDING AGENT
- Debriding agent of choice
- Dressing as indicated
- Petroleum jelly (optional)

Procedure

Surgical excision
1. Pick up the edge of the tissue with the forceps.

2. Cut necrotic tissue with the scissors or scalpel, leaving a margin of 0.5 cm to avoid cutting viable tissue.
3. Control bleeding by direct pressure.
4. After the procedure apply a sterile dressing. (See Wound care procedure.)

Topical debriding agents

1. Apply chemical agents to the gauze on the wound.
2. Allow the gauze to dry.
3. Pull off the gauze and debrided tissue as the dressing is changed.

Practitioners can apply enzyme preparations as a moist dressing. Use an occlusive dressing to retain the warmth and moisture essential for enzyme action.

It is important that the chemical agents and enzyme preparations not be applied to healthy tissue. Practitioners can protect the skin by using petroleum jelly on the healthy skin.

Hygroscopic dressings can also be used to debride necrotic tissue.

1. Apply the dressing.
2. Leave the dressing in place for 3 to 5 days.
3. Remove the dressing and the debrided tissue.

Hygroscopic dressings can be safely applied to healthy tissue.

For a more detailed list of specific agents see the article by Davis in the reference section. See Procedure for wound care.

Postprocedure patient education

Instruct the patient regarding wound care.

Instruct the patient regarding prevention of reoccurrence—hygiene, well-fitting shoes.

Practitioner Followup/Complications

The underlying causes of the ulcer must be treated.
Practitioners follow up for wound healing.
Practitioners monitor for infection, bleeding.
The use of systemic antibiotics should be considered.

CPT BILLING CODES

11040—Debridement; skin, partial thickness.

11041—Skin, full thickness.

11042—Skin and subcutaneous tissue.

11043—Skin, subcutaneous tissue, and muscle.

BIBLIOGRAPHY

Black JM, Black SB: Surgical management of pressure ulcers, *Nurs Clin North Am* 22(2):429, 1987.

Fowler EM: Equipment and products used in management and treatment of pressure ulcers, *Nurs Clin North Am* 22(2):449, 1987.

Honde C, Derks C, Tudor D: Local treatment of pressure sores in the elderly: amino acid copolymer membrane versus hydrocolloid dressing, *J Am Geriatr Soc* 42(11):1180, 1994.

Levine JM, Totolos E: Pressure ulcers: a strategic plan to prevent and heal them, *Geriatrics* 50(1):32, 1995.

Melcher RE, Longe RL, Gelbarg AO: Pressure sores in the elderly. A systematic approach to management, *Postgrad Med* 83(1):299, 1988.

Panel for the Prediction and Prevention of Pressure Ulcers in Adults: *Pressure ulcers in adults: prediction and prevention,* Clinical practice guideline, number 3, AHCPR publication No. 92-0047. Rockville, MD, May 1992, Agency for Health Care Policy and Research, Public Health Service, U.S. Department of Health and Human Services.

Perez ED: Pressure ulcers: updated guideline for treatment and prevention, *Geriatrics* 48(1):39, 1993.

Treatment of pressure ulcers, *Med Lett Drugs Ther* 32(812):17, 1990.

Xakellis GC Jr, Garzone P: Pressure ulcers, *Am Fam Physician* 35(4):159, 1987.

Yarkony GM: Pressure ulcers: a review, *Arch Phys Med Rehabil* 75(8):908, 1994.

Wound Care

Description

A moist wound bed promotes healing. Aseptic technique is used to minimize bacterial contamination.

Indications

Office treatment is indicated for minor wounds such as skin tears, first and minor second degree burns, and superficial lacerations. (Refer to Suturing procedure to evaluate need for sutures.)

Contraindications/Precautions

Wounds that require special caution occur in:

- Elderly patients with poor psychosocial support or concomitant disease
- Children who are less than 2 years old
- Conditions that predispose a patient to infection, such as diabetes, corticosteroid therapy, or immunodeficiency

Chemical, electrical, explosion, inhalation, or abuse-related injuries should be referred to an emergency room because of the extensive care required.

Practitioners assess iodine and sulfa drug allergies before starting treatment.

Patient Preparation/Education

Patients who call should be told that, before they visit the office, they should cover the wound with a clean, soft dressing.

Patients should be told not to apply ointments, butter, greases, or other compounds.

Equipment

- Gloves
- Normal saline
- 4 × 4 gauze
- Topical antibacterial agent: 1% silver sulfadiazine (burns)
- Tongue blade (burns)
- Choice of dressing:

  Semipermeable film (Op Site)
  Hydrocolloid (DuoDerm)
  Nonadherent gauze dressing (Telfa) and Kling (various sizes)

- Tape
- Tetanus toxoid (as indicated)

Procedure

1. Clean the wound using sterile normal saline or bland soap and water.
2. For burns, apply 1% silver sulfadiazine with a sterile tongue blade or a gloved hand, approximately 1/16-inch thick. If the patient is allergic to sulfa drugs, use a povidone–iodine ointment.
3. Apply nonadherent dressing (Telfa).
4. Wrap with gauze dressing (Kling) in layers, forming a soft bulky dressing, and secure with tape.
5. Tetanus toxoid 0.5 cc IM is given in the deltoid if the patient has not received a booster in the past 5 years.
6. Consider analgesic or antibiotic as indicated.
7. For semipermeable and hydrocolloid dressings:

   Dry the skin around the wound with a sterile 4 × 4 gauze.
   Apply the dressing according to the package directions.
   No cover dressing is necessary.

Postprocedure patient education

Instruct the patient with a Telfa dressing to provide daily wound care: Clean with sterile normal saline, apply antibiotic cream, and redress. Tell the patient to return to the office in 3 to 5 days.

Instruct patients with semipermeable films and hydrocolloids to leave the dressing on for 3 to 5 days, then return to the provider.

Advise patients to notify you if signs of infection occur (erythema, purulent drainage, odor, increase in pain, elevated temperature).

Practitioner Followup/Complications

The patient should be seen in 3 to 5 days.

To assess for signs of infection practitioners look for redness, swelling, blisters, drainage, and fever.

The patient should be referred to a physician if the wound is not healing.

BIBLIOGRAPHY

Agran MS, Engel MA, Mertz PM: Collagenase during burn wound healing: influence of a hydrogel dressing and pulsed electrical stimulation, *Plast Reconstr Surg* 94(3):518, 1994.

Coren CV: Burn injuries in children, *Pediatr Ann* 10(49):329, 1993.

David J: *Wound management: a comprehensive guide to dressing and healing*, Springhouse, Penn, 1986, Springhouse Corporation.

Gursel E, Binns J: Early management of burned patients, *Emerg Med Clin North Am* 1:595, 1983.

Parker G, Rendell E: Wound care. Hungry healers, *Nurs Times* 90(24):55, 1994.

Sieggreen M: Healing of physical wounds, *Nurs Clin North Am* 22(2):439, 1987.

Smith DJ, and others: Burn wounds: infection and healing, *Am J Surg* 167(1A):46S, 1994.

Tierney L, and others: *Current medical diagnosis & treatment*, Norwalk, Conn, 1992, Appleton & Lange.

Fungal Scraping—The KOH Test

Description

Superficial fungal infections of the skin, hair, and nails are commonly encountered in primary care. Scaling is a common characteristic of the disease process. These disorders result from infection of the skin by fungal organisms collectively called dermatophytes. Dermatophytes are keratinophilic (feed on keratin) and live primarily in the stratum corneum, hair, and nails. Fungal scraping of the skin is necessary to identify the causative organism.

The Wood's lamp shines an ultraviolet light. Certain fungal infections will fluoresce when viewed under the light of the Wood's lamp.

Indications

Fungal infection can manifest itself as scaly patches or a boggy inflammatory mass, patches of hair loss, or small scattered pustules. The physical findings and differential diagnosis will vary depending upon the location of the infection (Table 2-6). Children may have a fungal infection of the hair in which the hair is broken off at the skin level. This is called "black dot" tinea. The lesions may be very pruritic to the patient or barely noticeable. Therefore, if fungal infection is suspected, scrape.

Table 2-6

Differential Diagnosis

Name	Differential diagnosis
Tinea capitis (scalp)	Alopecia areata Seborrheic dermatitis Pyoderma
Tinea corporis (body)	Nummular eczema Pityriasis rosea (herald patch) Psoriasis Impetigo
Tinea cruris (groin)	Intertrigo Candidiasis
Tinea pedis (feet)	Hyperhidrosis Dry skin Contact dermatitis Dyshidrotic eczema
Tinea manuum (hand)	Contact dermatitis Psoriasis
Tinea faciale (face)	Photodermatitis Lupus erythematosus Seborrheic dermatitis
Tinea unguium (nail)	Psoriasis Trauma
Tinea versicolor (trunk)	Vitiligo (white) Seborrheic dermatitis (tan or pink)

Complications are rare, and secondary bacterial infections are uncommon. Fungal infections can sometimes produce pustules (especially around hair follicles), and the examiner may misdiagnose these pustules as bacterial in origin. Kerions, which present as tender, edematous, erythematous lesions, may be mistaken for bacterial infections. Kerions result from a hypersensitivity reaction to the tinea capitis and are treated by treating the fungal infection. Positive fungal scrapings would confirm the diagnosis. Certain tinea can gain access to deeper tissues and cause cellulitis of the lower extremities.

Contraindications/Precautions

Caution needs to be taken when scraping the suspected area with the instrument. The skin should not be broken open over the pustules, and the dermis or epidermis should not be cut accidentally with the edge of the scalpel, if one is used.

Patient Preparation/Education

Practitioners explain to the patient that this is a painless, quick, and noninvasive procedure.

Patients should be asked whether they have already tried treating the skin lesion with an antifungal agent, as that could interfere with obtaining accurate results.

Equipment

- Soft bristle toothbrush, No. 15 scalpel, or wooden tongue depressor
- One glass microscope slide and 1 plastic cover slip
- Microscope with 10× objective
- 10% or 20% potassium hydroxide (KOH) solution
- Heat source (match, alcohol lamp, or cigarette lighter)
- Forceps (optional, for hair)
- Wood's lamp (optional)

Procedure

1. Scrape the edge of the lesion where there are fine scales. Avoid thick scales. If there is hair loss, sample the short, broken hairs with the scalpel, or use the forceps to pluck the hair. If the nail is involved, scrape thin pieces of nail.
2. Place the samples on the slide, using the scalpel blade to gather the scales without overlapping to the center of the slide.
3. Place 1 or 2 drops of KOH solution on the sample. Warning: KOH is very caustic; therefore avoid contact with skin and eyes. It may cause permanent damage to microscope objectives and other equipment.
4. Place a coverslip over the specimen. Use plastic coverslips so that

loose scales are picked up by the electrostatic charge to the underside.

5. Gently heat the slide over the heat source. An alcohol lamp is preferable as it does not leave any black carbon on the undersurface of the slide. Avoid boiling the slide contents; the bottom of the slide should feel quite warm to the touch. Heat serves to speed the chemical reaction of KOH dissolving the keratin of the scales. Allow skin scrapings to stand for about 5 minutes. Hair must sit for 15 to 30 minutes. Nails must sit for 30 minutes.

6. Place the slide on the microscope and examine it under low light on 10× magnification. The refractile quality of the fungus hyphae are more pronounced under the low light. Scan the entire field for the thin, long, branched forms of the hyphae, which may or may not be accompanied by spores. When an object is found that looks suspicious, examine it under a higher power (250× magnification) to look for internal structures such as vacuoles. Cell walls have an irregular linearity, whereas threads appear uniform and lack internal structure.

7. To examine with the Wood's lamp, darken the room and shine the Wood's lamp on skin at a distance of 8 inches from skin.

Interpretation of results

A positive KOH test occurs when hyphae are visualized. See Figure 2-14 for the characteristic appearance of hyphae.

A positive Wood's lamp test occurs when the skin fluoresces:

Tinea capitis—yellow green to pale green
Tinea versicolor—golden yellow
Dermatophytosis in the hair shaft—green to yellow

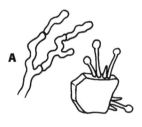
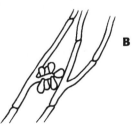

Fig. 2-14 Characteristic appearance of hyphae. **A** *Trichophyton verruscosum.* **B** *Trichophyton interdigitale.*

Erythrasma (caused by *Corynebacterium minutissimum*)—coral red

Other substances may also fluoresce, such as tetracycline, fluorescein dye, and many cosmetics.

Postprocedure patient education

Instruct patients on how to use the antifungal medication prescribed.

Instruct patient about hygiene that discourages further fungal infections (keep skin clean and dry, avoid walking on locker room floors in bare feet, use cotton socks and underwear, etc).

Practitioner Followup/Complications

If the KOH test is positive, treatment with oral or topical antifungals is necessary.

The practitioner may reevaluate the patient in 2 or 3 days by telephone to see whether there has been improvement, or the patient can be instructed to call the office if the signs and symptoms are not improving. If the infection does not improve in a few days (or a few weeks in the case of tinea capitis), the patient should come back for reevaluation of the diagnosis.

If the KOH test is inconclusive, the practitioner may elect to do a culture of the lesion using DTM (dermatophyte test medium). It will take 3 to 5 days to culture out, but the results are highly reliable and easy to read (look for a characteristic color change of the medium from yellow to bright red and fluffy white colonies of dermatophytes—fungi). The disadvantage is that normal flora of *Candida* (not necessarily an infection) will also give a positive result.

Fungal infections can get secondary bacterial infections, but this is very rare.

BIBLIOGRAPHY

Goldgeier MH: Fungal infections of the skin, hair and nails, *Pediatr Ann* 22(4):253, 1993.
Pariser DM: Diagnostic and therapeutic techniques for evaluation and treatment of skin disorders, *Primary Care* 16:823, 1989.
Pariser DM: Superficial fungal infections. A practical guide for primary care physicians, *Postgrad Med* 87(5):205, 1990.
Taplin D, Meinking TL: Scabies, lice, and fungal infections, *Primary Care* 16(3):551, 1989.

Tick Removal

Description

Ticks are becoming more frequently encountered in primary care. The importance of prompt, proper tick removal has increased with the advent of Lyme disease. Rocky Mountain spotted fever remains endemic in many areas of the United States.

Lyme disease is caused by the spirochete *Borrelia burgdorferi*. Lyme disease is transmitted by the ixodid or smaller deer tick. The female deer tick is about 2 to 3 mm long, with a red body and black legs. Rocky Mountain spotted fever (RMSF) is caused by *Rickettsia rickettsii* and is transmitted by the larger dog tick.

Indications

Ticks attached to the body need to be removed as soon as possible.

Contraindications/Precautions

If a tick is removed within 24 hours the chance of transmission of Lyme disease is greatly decreased.

It is important not to squeeze the body of the tick when removing it because squeezing will push fluid from the tick into the human.

Applying hot matches or noxious chemicals to the tick is contraindicated.

Equipment

- Fine tipped tweezers
- Alcohol wipe
- Betadine swab
- Bottle with alcohol for saving tick (optional)

Procedure

1. Clean the area with an alcohol wipe.
2. Grab the tick at a point of attachment (mouth), not by the body of the tick.
3. Pull firmly, but with gentle traction. Do not twist or crush.
4. Put the tick in a bottle with alcohol if its identification is desired.
5. Clean the area with Betadine.

Postprocedure patient education

Warn patients that people who live in or visit an area where ticks are common should check the skin every evening for ticks. Suggest that partners can check each other in places that are difficult to check, such as scalp and back.

Instruct patients that ticks can be better avoided by wearing protective clothing and using repellents.

Tell the patient to watch for the symptoms of Lyme disease: erythema migrans (a flat or slightly raised red lesion that expands with central clearing); other secondary lesions; a flulike illness with fever, chills, and myalgia; headache or stiff neck; and arthralgia. Erythema migrans occurs in 60% to 80% of cases. Lyme disease can be found anywhere in the continental United States; however most cases are found in the north eastern coastal states, the upper midwest, and northern California.

Inform the patient that the presentation of Rocky Mountain spotted fever is usually fever, malaise, severe frontal headache, myalgias, and vomiting. The rash, when present, appears as macules on the wrists and ankles, then spreads to the trunk, face, palms, and sole. Papules, petechia, and purpura may develop. RMSF may be found across the United States, but is predominantly found in the south Atlantic costal states and the western and south central states.

Practitioner Followup/Complications

Usually no followup is necessary.

Uncomplicated bites can be painful and leave a red puncture wound that takes 1 to 2 weeks to heal.

The most frequent complication is infection of the area, which is usually prevented by cleaning the area with betadine.

Rarely, bites cause a delayed hypersensitivity reaction, with fever, pruritus, and urticaria.

A granuloma can develop if a tick is removed improperly, leaving tick parts in the skin. If a firm, pruritic, red papule or nodule persists, removal by a surgeon may be necessary.

CPT BILLING CODE

10120—Removal of superficial foreign body, skin.

BIBLIOGRAPHY

Middleton DB: Tick-borne infections, *Postgrad Med* 95(5):131, 1994.
Spach DH, and others: Tick-borne diseases in the United States, *NEJM* 329(13):936, 1993.
Tierney LM, McPhee SJ, Papadakis MA: *Current Medical Diagnosis & Treatment,* Norwalk, Conn, 1994, Appleton & Lange.

Corn and Callus Management

Description

A callus represents the gradual development of a thickened stratum corneum in a localized area of tissue, resulting from continued physical trauma. Common causes include friction from poorly fitting shoes along the inner aspects of the sole, heel, and great toe, and on the distal digit of the fingers from the pressure of holding a pencil or pen; any area exposed to repeated friction and pressure may be affected.

Corns are hyperkeratotic lesions present over bony prominences and involving the stratum corneum or horny layer of the skin. A corn is either soft or hard and is caused by pressure secondary to an unyielding structure.

With a hard corn, the phalangeal condyle under the skin and an unyielding shoe over the skin generates pressure and friction. A painful lesion develops over the dorsolateral aspect of the proximal interphalangeal joint of the fifth toe. The lesion is firm, dry, and tender and can have surrounding erythema and heat present if acutely irritated. A bursa may even develop. Hard corn removal usually requires surgical resection and should be referred to a podiatrist.

The soft corn is usually interdigital and the most common place is the fourth web space. It is caused by pressure imposed by the lateral side of the base of the fourth proximal phalanx, the medial condyle of the head of the fifth proximal phalanx, or both.

Most calluses and corns may be treated conservatively. Problems that are more extensive require minor surgical intervention by a podiatrist or surgeon. It is the minor, conservative treatment that is discussed here.

Indications

Indications for removing corns and calluses are pain, swelling, and redness that hinders the patient's ambulation or ability to wear shoes.

Contraindications/Precautions

Practitioners should proceed cautiously in diabetic or immunocompromised patients.

Corns that are deeply imbedded, extensive in nature, or extend into the nail bed should be referred.

Hard corns may require resection of head and neck of proximal phalanx and should be referred to a podiatrist.

Patient Preparation/Education

Patients should soak their feet in warm water for 20 minutes the night before the procedure to soften tissue.

The skin may be scrubbed with a pumice stone to remove any loose tissue.

The feet may be soaked again before the procedure.

Equipment

- Lamb's wool or self-adherent web spacer

- No. 15 scalpel
- Pumice stone, sanding board, or electric burr

Procedure

For removal of hard or soft corns

1. Instruct the patient to wash toes and web spaces twice a day with household soap, dry completely, and apply an antifungal, antibacterial powder and a lamb's wool or self-adherent rubber web spacer (doughnut; may be found in a foot care section in a retail store).
2. Instruct the patient to use over-the-counter salicylate pads, which soften the tissue, continuously for 7–10 days. Remove the pads and debride with a pumice stone, rubbing deeply to remove the firm inner core. A scalpel may be used to remove this core.

Postprocedure patient education

Instruct the patient to keep the toes dressed for 3 weeks, in proper position, followed by 3 weeks of taping the toes together loosely with lamb's wool between them.

Tell the patient to report any signs of infection (redness, increased pain, swelling, warmth, foul smelling discharge) at once.

Procedure

For removal of calluses

1. Use a sanding board, pumice stone, or electric burr to thin and smooth any thick or rough calluses.
2. Proceed slowly so that a firm intact layer of skin remains after sanding.
3. A scalpel can be used to slice off layers of very thick calluses.

Postprocedure patient education

Instruct the patient to try to remove the source of irritation to prevent the recurrence of calluses.

Practitioner Followup/Complications

Practitioners should evaluate the patient within 1 week for signs of infection and the extent of healing.

CPT BILLING CODES

11050-11052—Paring or curettement of benign hyperkeratotic skin lesion with or without chemical cauterization (such as verrucae or clavi) not extending through the stratum corneum (e.g., callus or wart) with or without local anesthesia; single lesion.

BIBLIOGRAPHY

Helfand AE: Nail and hyperkeratotic problems in the elderly foot, *Am Fam Physician* 39(2):101, 1989.
Klenerman L, ed: *The foot and its disorders,* ed 3, London, 1991, Mosby.
Pfenninger JL, Fowler GC: *Procedures for primary care physicians,* St Louis, 1994, Mosby.
Richardson EG: *Campbell's operative orthopaedics,* vol 4, St Louis, 1992, Mosby.

Toenail Care in the Diabetic Patient

Description

This procedure describes the routine care of nails in diabetic patients. The procedure is also indicated for other patients with chronic diseases that impair circulation. Foot infections and their direct sequelae are the complications of diabetes that most frequently lead to hospitalization. The consequences of foot ulceration include extensive human suffering, prolonged functional disability, increased risk of amputation, and associated mortality. It is estimated that more than 50% of the nontraumatic amputations in the United States occur in diabetic patients and that, within this population, more than 50% can be prevented by improved foot care.

Indications

The prevention of foot infections in a person with diabetes requires proper foot care by the patient as well as early detection and prompt treatment by the health care provider. Figure 2-15 (p. 85) illustrates the anatomy of the toenail.

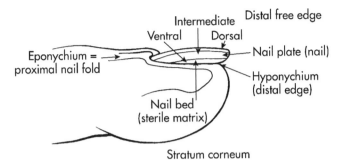

Fig. 2-15 Nail bed anatomy and terminology. (From Pfenninger JL, Fowler GC: *Procedures for primary care physicians,* St Louis, 1994, Mosby.)

The provider should perform the foot care whenever the patient is unable to perform foot and nail care, or when the patient has a nail or foot condition that cannot be safely managed by the patient.

The need for care is obvious when the toenails are excessively long, rough, or thick; when nails present the risk of injury to the patient from the nails or trauma to the nails themselves; when there is inflammation, infection, or injury in the nails or feet; or when excessive corns or calluses cause pain or pressure.

Contraindications/Precautions

Neuropathy, vascular insufficiency, and an altered response to infection make the diabetic patient susceptible to foot infections. The prevention of foot infections in a patient with diabetes requires routine foot care.

To avoid burns, do not use an electric burr on a patient whose foot cannot be held still.

The practitioner should refer the patient to a podiatrist when the nail is very deformed or the patient is acutely ill with diabetes mellitus, peripheral neuropathy, blood dyscrasias, peripheral vascular disease, or being managed on steroids.

Patient Preparation/Education

Unless inflammation or infection is present, it is preferable to soak the feet in warm water or wrap the feet in a warm, damp washcloth for about 10 minutes before the procedure.

Practitioners should instruct the patient that the procedure should not hurt.

Equipment

- Clippers or scissor. Concave nail clippers of the plier type can be purchased in a medical supply store.
- Pumice stone (medium sandpaper may be more affordable for some patients).
- Emery board or electric burr (sander).

Procedure

1. Inspect the nails, the foot, and between the toes for color changes, calluses, blisters, cracks, cuts, bruises, ingrown nails, ulcers, or signs of infection.
2. Check for warmth of extremity and pulses.
3. Always trim toenails straight across. Cut nails with clippers in small snips rather than attempting to cut an entire nail in one stroke.
4. Don't cut the nail so short as to cause bleeding. It should not be cut below the top of the toe. Cut nail edges in slightly rounded fashion for smoothness, but do not cut at sharp down angles at corners (Fig. 2-16).
5. File any remaining sharp edges with an emery board. Smooth the edges and thin the undersides of thickened nails with a sanding board or electric burr. Thick fungal nails are best managed with thinning and shaping rather than treating.
6. Buff calluses or corns lightly with a pumice stone or sandpaper to prevent cracking and breaks in the skin integrity.
7. Do not disturb the cuticles because they provide barriers against infection.

Postprocedure patient education

All individuals with diabetes should learn the principles of foot self-examination and care. Inform the patients of why this is so im-

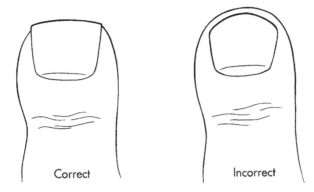

Fig. 2-16 Proper nail care prophylaxis. Trim the nail flat but not too short. (From Pfenninger JL, Fowler GC: *Procedures for primary care physicians,* St Louis, 1994, Mosby.)

portant and instruct them to observe the procedure closely so it can be repeated at home. Give patients the following instructions:

- The best time to trim nails is following a bath or shower when the nails are softer.
- Keep toenails trimmed.
- Keep feet and nails clean.
- Never treat calluses, blisters, ingrown nails or wounds at home; it can lead to serious infection. Contact the health care provider.
- Ingrown nails are often caused by tight-fitting shoes or incorrect nail trimming. Shoes must fit well with room for toes.
- Signs of infection (color change, warmth, inflammation, tenderness if sensation is intact, drainage). Contact the health care provider if any occur.
- Inspect the feet every day because decreased sensation may prevent the usual alarm symptom of tenderness. Use a mirror to inspect the bottoms of the feet if necessary.
- Do not dig into the corners of toenails with sharp objects because it may injure the delicate nail fold and may lead to infection.
- Visit the health care provider regularly and be sure the feet are examined at each visit.

If a dressing has been applied because of an open area, then teach the patient wound care.

Practitioner Followup/Complications

Localized infection may develop in patients with poor circulation or when the procedure is not gently performed.

CPT BILLING CODES

11700—Debridement of nails, manual; five or less.
11701—Each additional, five or less.
11710—Debridement of nails, electric grinder; five or less.
11711—Each additional, five or less.

BIBLIOGRAPHY

Christensen MH, and others: How to care for the diabetic foot, *Am J Nurs* 91:50, 1991.
Helfand AE: Nail and hyperkeratotic problems in the elderly foot, *Am Fam Physician,* 39(2):101, 1989.
Klenerman L, ed: *The foot and its disorders,* ed 3, London, 1991, Mosby.
Kozak G, and others, eds: *Management of diabetic foot problems,* ed 2, Philadelphia, 1995, WB Saunders.
Leichter SB, Schaefer JC, O'Brien JT: New concepts in managing diabetic foot infections, *Geriatrics,* 46(5):24, 1991.
Lipsky BA, Pecoraro RE, Ahroni JH: Foot ulceration and infections in elderly diabetics, *Clin Geriatr Med* 6:747, 1990.
Lipsky BA, Pecoraro RE, Wheat L: The diabetic foot: soft tissue and bone infection, *Infect Dis Clin North Am* 4(3):409, 1990.
Physician's guide to non-insulin dependent (type II) diabetes: diagnosis and treatment, ed 2, Alexandria, 1988, American Diabetic Association.

Ingrown Toenail Management

Description

Ingrown toenails are a common problem and can cause significant pain and disability. Shoes that are too tight or toenails that are improperly cut can cause the painful swelling, redness, and tenderness around the corner of the toenail on the great toe. Toe nail removal, either partial or total, is the procedure indicated for conditions in which a spur or splinter of nail has invaded the sulcus and subsequent subcutaneous tissue (onychocryptosis). As the splinter portion of nail continues to grow within the sulcus, inflammation in the surrounding tissue occurs (paronychia).

Three stages of ingrown toenails have been described. The first is characterized by redness, pain, and slight swelling; the second by swelling, pain, and redness with infection and suppuration; and the third by granulation tissue formation and hypertrophy of the nail wall, with all the characteristics of the second stage more pronounced. Stage I and II ingrown toenails can be successfully treated with conservative management or partial nail removal as described in this procedure. Stage III ingrown toenails are better treated with more aggressive, surgical procedures under local anesthesia and should be referred to the proper specialist.

Indications

The following conditions need treatment and management:

- Onychocryptosis (ingrown nail)
- Onychomycosis (fungal infection of the nail)
- Chronic, recurrent paronychia
- Onychogryposis (deformed, curved nail)

Contraindications/Precautions

A history of allergy to local anesthetics is a contraindication. The presence of bleeding diathesis is also a contraindication.

Patient Preparation/Education

The patient should soak the affected toe(s) in an antiseptic–germicidal solution for about 15 to 20 minutes. This may be done during the patient education time or while preparing for the minor surgical procedure.

Before the procedure the patient should be instructed to wear open-toed shoes, such as sandals, because of postoperative bandages.

Practitioners should inform the patient that ill-fitting shoes need to be replaced with properly fitted shoes.

Practitioners should explain the procedure sufficiently to assure the cooperation of the patient or caregiver because home treatment for several weeks is required.

Equipment

CONSERVATIVE MANAGEMENT

- Antiseptic–germicidal solution and a pan for soaking toe(s)
- Gloves
- Scissors to trim nail edge
- Nail file
- Nail elevator
- Cotton for packing and protection
- Antibiotic ointment (optional)

PARTIAL NAIL REMOVAL

- Antiseptic–germicidal solution and pan for soaking toe(s)
- Gloves
- Anesthetic without epinephrine (see Anesthesia procedure)
- Betadine
- Tourniquet—Penrose drain (optional)
- Nail elevator
- Nail splitter
- Forceps
- Beaver blade
- Hemostat
- Curette
- Phenol (optional)
- Antibiotic ointment
- Sterile bandage and tape

Procedure

Conservative management

1. Once the nail is softened and cleaned, cut off the offending nail corner.
2. Then thin the middle one-third of the nail (10 to 15 mm) by filing the upper surface until the nail matrix can be seen beneath.
3. Elevate the nail edge and remove any debris or infected material. Minimal amounts of granulation tissue can be reduced by application of silver nitrate.

4. Pack a small piece of cotton firmly under the nail edge. Cotton wool soaked in 60% alcohol may also be used.
5. If the cuticle is swollen or infected, apply an antibiotic ointment before packing.
6. If the medial edge of the toenail is involved, protect it by taping cotton between the first and second toes to keep them from touching.
7. If the lateral edge is involved, protect it by taping the cotton to the outside of the ball of the toe which keeps the toenail from touching the inside of the shoe.

Partial nail removal
1. Position the patient comfortably in a supine or semirecumbent position.
2. Administer a bilateral digital nerve block with 2% lidocaine (without epinephrine). The purpose is to block sensory fibers of the dorsal and plantar digital nerves (see Anesthesia procedure).
3. Clean the toe with an antiseptic solution such as Betadine.
4. Apply tourniquet (optional). Some use the tourniquet to decrease bleeding and maintain a more localized anesthesia.
5. Use the nail elevator to free the nail sulcus and eponychium from the nail plate.
6. Split a 2- to 3-mm wedge of nail with the nail splitter.
7. Push the beaver blade under the eponychium to free the remainder of the nail.
8. Remove the wedged section using the hemostat by carefully rotating the separated portion toward the remainder of the healthy nail plate (Fig. 2-17, p. 92). This separates any buried portion of the nail and prevents embedding of a spicule of nail. The distalmost portion of the nail will have a feather look if it has been removed intact.
9. Curet the matrix and nail bed to remove any missed nail and additional debris.
10. Apply phenol to cauterize and destroy that part of the matrix from which the wedge has been removed (optional). In the absence of phenol, growth of new nail takes approximately 8 to 12 months in an adult.

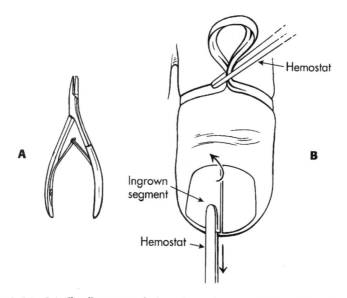

Fig. 2-17 A Nail splitter. **B** Technique for nail removal after nail has been split. Grasp that portion of the nail to be removed lengthwise with a straight hemostat, and remove it using a steady pulling motion with a simultaneous upward twist of the hand toward the affected side. (From Pfenninger JL, Fowler GC: *Procedures for primary care physicians,* St Louis, 1994, Mosby.)

11. Remove tourniquet.
12. Apply an antibiotic ointment such as Bacitracin to a piece of Owens silk or similar medium to the surgical area. Apply sterile 2 × 2 gauze and wrap with a self-adhesive tape.

Postprocedure patient education

Give the patient the following instructions:

- Rest the foot and keep it elevated for 12 to 24 hours.
- Remove the bandage the night after surgery and soak the foot 5 to 10 minutes in plain warm water, never hot. If there is difficulty removing the bandage for the initial soak, place the entire bandage into the water for 5 to 10 minutes to allow it to come off more easily.
- Soak the toe 10 to 15 minutes 2 times a day in an antiseptic–germicidal solution or a 1:120 bleach solution (a tablespoon of bleach per 2 quarts of water with a little liquid soap) for cleaning and killing germs.

- During the soaks, massage the swollen part of the cuticle outward and bend the corners of the offending nail upward.
- After soaking, dry the foot and cover the nail bed with an antibiotic ointment.
- Reapply the cotton packing, if used, after each soaking.
- Then cover with a bandage.
- Watch for any red streaks up the foot or leg, fever or chills, or warmth and pain. If these signs are present, call the practitioner immediately.
- Normally, there will be a small amount of drainage for 1 to 2 weeks after surgery.
- If the cuticle becomes swollen or infected (oozes pus or other secretions), triple antibiotic ointment should be applied 5 to 6 times a day.
- Wearing sandals or going barefoot (where it is safe to do so) will prevent continued pressure on the toenail. When closed-toed shoes are worn, be sure there is plenty of room in the toes and protect the offending toe(s) from further injury with cotton padding.

Prevention

Practitioners should give the patient these instructions:

- Ingrown toe nails are most frequently a result of incorrect cutting of nails. Never cut the nail so short that part of the nail bed is exposed. The free edge should be cut straight across. Direct the growth of the nail over the cuticle edge instead of into it.
- Excessive pressure on the nails caused by wearing tight shoes or constrictive hosiery, even for as short a time as 1 week, may also lead to ingrown or imbedded nails.

Practitioner Followup/Complications

Practitioners should watch for infection.

Practitioners should evaluate for regrowth of the nail and the return of symptoms.

An upward-turned deformity of the distal nail bed and pulp may develop as a result of therapy.

The patient's nail is to be rechecked in 1 to 2 weeks following surgery, or sooner if there are signs and symptoms of infection.

Prophylactic antibiotics [e.g., cephalexin (Keflex) 250 to 500 mg qid × 7 days] are prescribed in a patient with compromised health.

If symptoms persist despite treatment, refer the patient to a podiatrist.

CPT BILLING CODES

11730-11750—Avulsion of nail plate, partial or complete.

BIBLIOGRAPHY

Connolly B, Fitzgerald RJ: Pledgets in ingrowing toenails, *Arch Dis Child* 63(1):71, 1988.

Krull MD, Neale EA, Adams IM, editors: *Common food disorders,* ed 3, New York, 1989, Churchill Livingstone.

Ilfeld FW: Ingrown toenail treated with cotton collodion insert, *Foot & Ankle* 11(5):312, 1991.

Murray WR: Management of ingrowing toenail, *Br J Surg* 76(9):883, 1989.

Reijnen JAM, Goris RJA: Conservative treatment of ingrowing toenails, *Br J Surg* 76(9):955, 1989.

Richardson EG: *Campbell's operative orthopaedics,* St Louis, 1992, Mosby.

Scher RK, Daniel CR, editors: *Nails: therapy, diagnosis, surgery,* Philadelphia, 1990, WB Saunders.

Schmidt BD: Toenail, Ingrown. In *Instructions for pediatric patients,* Philadelphia, 1992, WB Saunders.

Seigle RJ, Stewart R: Recalcitrant ingrown nails: surgical approaches, *J Dermatol Surg Oncol* 18(8):744, 1992.

Sykes PA, Kerr R: Treatment of ingrowing toenails by surgeons and chiropodists, *BMJ* 297(6644):335, 1988.

van der Ham AC, Hackeng CA, Yo TI: The treatment of ingrowing toenails. A randomised comparison of wedge excision and phenol cauterization, *J Bone Joint Surg,* 72(3):507, 1990.

Subungual Hematoma Evacuation

Description

Trauma to the fingernail or toenail can cause bleeding between the nail bed and the nail. The resulting subungual hematoma—a swelling or mass of blood confined beneath the nail caused by broken blood vessels—slowly expands over several hours, resulting in persistent, often throbbing, pain. Causes other than trauma include systemic pathology, medications, drug reactions, or aging. The hematoma can be recognized, usually, by a blue-black or blue-purple area under the nail at the site of the trauma that is exquisitely and increasingly more painful. Drainage of the accumulated blood in the hematoma (decompression of the hematoma) usually brings immediate relief of the pain. This procedure minimizes the possibility of secondary pressure effects to the digit and dystrophy of the nail bed and matrix and is required to prevent unnecessary delay in regrowth of the nail plate.

Indications

This procedure is indicated for visible, painful subungual hematomas involving less than 25% of the nail bed.

Contraindications/Precautions

If the nail is crushed or fractured, the patient should be referred to a specialist.

If the phalanx is fractured, the patient should be referred to a specialist.

If a subungual melanoma (a malignant pigmented tumor beneath the nail) is present, the patient should be referred to a specialist.

Hematomas involving greater than 50% of the nail may indicate laceration of the underlying nail bed. The practitioner should consider referral to a specialist for removal of the entire nail.

Patient Preparation/Education

This procedure usually does not hurt any more than what the patient is already experiencing.

A slightly irritating or bad smell may occur.

Equipment

- Gloves
- Betadine or other antiseptic–germicidal solution
- Alcohol wipe

- No. 11 scalpel, hot paper clip, cautery, or 18-gauge needle
- Lighter to heat paper clip
- Sterile gauze
- Antibiotic ointment
- Bandage
- Splint (if necessary)

Procedure

1. Examine the injured digit to determine the extent of injury. Using your thumb and index finger, gently squeeze the lateral and medial sides of the proximal interphalangeal joint. If this area is pain free, there is probably no extensive fracture beyond the terminal tuft. The examiner may then proceed distally to determine whether a more extensive fracture is possible. If the examiner suspects a nondisplaced fracture, apply a splint in an anatomic (slightly curved) position until the swelling has decreased.
2. Radiographs of the involved digits are recommended to detect associated distal phalangeal fractures (terminal tuft fracture) when there is a reasonable index of suspicion.
3. Soak the affected digit in antiseptic solution during the patient education time and/or while preparing for the procedure.
4. Clean the nail with alcohol.
5. Using an 18-gauge needle or a No. 11 scalpel blade, and using a rotary motion, bore a hole through the nail to the hematoma.
6. Alternatively, burn a small hole in the nail using a conventional hand-held cautery or with the straightened end of a paper clip. Heat the straightened portion of the paper clip with a lighter until the tip is red hot. Apply the hot tip with gentle pressure to the nail over the site of the hematoma (Fig. 2-18).
7. Repeat step 6 two or three times. A small hole will be slowly burned through the nail. Make sure the hole is large enough to allow drainage. A sudden burst of blood may occur if the pressure beneath the nail is great enough.
8. After the blood has been drained and pressure and pain relieved, clean the area once more with alcohol.

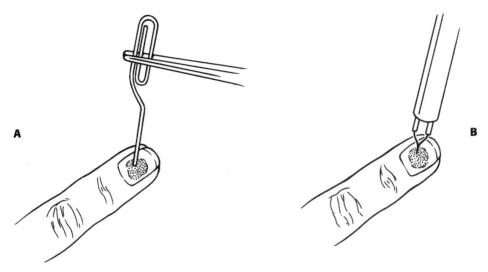

Fig. 2-18 A A heated paper clip is placed directly over the hematoma to perforate the nail. **B** A cautery unit may be used to perforate the nail and evacuate the subungual hematoma. (From Pfenninger JL, Fowler GC: *Procedures for primary care physicians,* St Louis, 1994, Mosby.)

9. Apply antibiotic ointment and a light dressing or adhesive strip to the nail.
10. The patient may use a splint for 2 or 3 days on an injured finger to protect it from further injury and pain.

Postprocedure patient education

Tell the patients to soak the affected digit two or three times a day and to keep a light dressing or adhesive strip over the area until the empty space has completely closed.

Instruct the patients to keep the injured extremity elevated as much as possible to reduce the swelling.

Instruct the patients to notify the practitioner if the pain persists, if drainage becomes purulent or foul smelling, or if there is a change in the sensation of the finger, a fever, or redness of the skin surrounding the injury.

Advise the patients that the nail should be feeling progressively better in a few days and if the bleeding returns, the pain worsens, or the injury is not getting better, they should call or come back.

If this procedure does not relieve the pain within a reasonable amount of time refer the patients to a podiatrist for further treatment.

Practitioner Followup/Complications

Practitioners watch for onycholysis (slow loosening of the nail from its bed, usually beginning at the free or loosened end and progressing to the root).

Practitioners check for transient or permanent nail deformity.

Practitioners evaluate for signs of infection.

CPT BILLING CODES

11740—Evacuation of subungual hematoma.

BIBLIOGRAPHY

Baran R, Haneke E: Surgery of the nail. In Epstein E, Epstein E, editors: *Skin Surgery,* ed 6, Philadelphia, 1987, WB Saunders.

Eisele SA: Conditions of the toenails, *Orthop Clin North Am* 25(1):183, 1994.

Fountain JA: Recognition of subungual hematoma as an imitator of subungual melanoma, *J Am Acad Dermatol* 23(4, Pt 1):773, 1990.

Grisafi PJ, and others: Three selected subungual pathologies: subungual exostosis, subungual osteochondroma, and subungual hematoma, *Clin Podiatr Med Surg* 6(2):355, 1989.

Helfand AE: Nail and hyperkeratotic problems in the elderly foot, *Am Fam Physician* 39(2):101, 1989.

Palamarchuk HJ, Kerzner M: An improved approach to evacuation of subungual hematoma, *J Am Podiatr Med Assn* 79(11):566, 1989.

Schwartz MW, editor: *Pediatric primary care: a problem oriented approach,* Chicago, 1990, Year–Book Medical Publishers, p. 654.

Stone OJ: Commonsense advice on treating nail disorders, *Postgrad Med* 85(6):279, 1989.

CHAPTER 3

Eye, Ear, and Nose Procedures

Removal of a Foreign Body from the Eye

Description

The most common ocular injury is caused by a simple foreign body. Corneal abrasions, erosion, or cuts produce the same symptoms as a foreign body in the eye. Not all foreign body injuries are associated with pain; glass embedded in the cornea may be particularly difficult to detect.

Common sites of foreign bodies in the eye are the conjunctival fornix of the upper lid, within the lid fissure, sunk into an angle of the anterior chamber inferiorly, within the posterior wall, or within the vitreous cavity.

Indications

Indications that a foreign body needs to be removed from the eye are:

- Unilateral foreign body sensation
- Red eye
- Eye trauma
- Unilateral eye irritation in contact lens wearers

99

A primary care provider can remove foreign bodies embedded in the conjunctival sac or in the corneal epithelium that are easily seen without magnification. Fluorescein staining will outline the area.

Contraindications/Precautions

Foreign bodies may serve as a focus for infection.

Practitioners do not use corticosteroids in the eye. Steroids can cause rapid activation of herpes, promote growth of fungi, potentiate the collagenolytic effect of enzymes of organisms such as *Pseudomonas*, and impair wound healing.

Iron or steel foreign bodies will frequently form ring-shaped orange stains that cause a low-grade inflammation and impair vision.

The eyeball should not be pressed against at any time.

The following should be referred to an ophthalmologist or emergency room:

- Injury in which intraocular damage is suspected because of the mechanism of injury (for example, small object propelled toward the eye, hammering metal, etc.)
- Blood in the anterior chamber of the eye
- Fixed, distorted, or dilated pupils
- Change in visual acuity
- Visible flecks of steel or iron surrounded by a rust ring
- Foreign body imbedded inside the eyeball or deeply lodged in the sclera or cornea
- Painless loss of vision
- Chemical or liquids in the eye (Immediate management is eye irrigation with normal saline or water for at least 15 minutes)
- Uncooperative patient (mentally deficient individual, a young child, or a demented adult)

Patient Preparation/Education

During an eye examination, the patient is usually frightened, upset, and apprehensive. If the patient has pain, he or she will keep the eye shut tightly as a defense mechanism. The patient will need reassurance, so explain each step of the procedure. Often a local topical anesthetic is required to permit adequate inspection of the eye. Explain that the anesthetic will take effect in about 1 minute but will not block sensation completely.

Equipment

- Bright light
- Snellen eye chart
- Sterile normal saline
- Topical anesthetic drops (proparacaine HCl 0.5%)
- Topical antimicrobial drops or ointment (sulfacetamide 10%)
- Eye spud or small-gauge needle (25 gauge)
- Fluorescein-impregnated strips
- Penlight or cobalt blue light
- Sterile cotton-tipped applicator
- Ophthalmoscope

Procedure

Preparation

1. Obtain a history (full description of the current episode, past relevant history, allergies, if the injury was employment related, etc.).
2. Check visual acuity.
3. If it is difficult for the patient to keep the eye open because of pain, instill 1 to 2 drops of 0.5% topical anesthetic and wait about 1 minute.

Examination

1. Inspect the cornea and sclera using a light source. Open the lids wide, using your thumb and index finger. If a foreign body is detected, use the removal technique for a particle before proceeding (see Removal techniques).
2. Apply fluorescein dye:
   a. Moisten the tip of a dye strip with sterile saline.
   b. Touch the strip to the conjunctiva. (If you are staining both eyes, use separate strips to prevent cross-contamination.)
   c. Instruct the patient to blink the eye gently and look straight ahead.

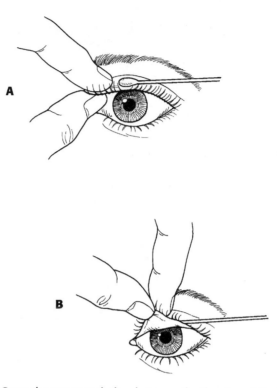

Fig. 3-1 **A** Grasp the upper eyelashes between the thumb and the index finger and, with the tip of the other index finger or a cotton-tipped applicator, press gently on the skin at the upper lateral border of the tarsal plate. **B** Pull outward on the lashes and rotate the tarsal plate upward until it forms a right angle with the eyeball. A gentle tug upward should flip the plate into eversion, clearly exposing the conjunctival surface of the upper lid. (From Pfenninger JL, Fowler GC: *Procedures for primary care physicians,* St Louis, 1994, Mosby.)

    d. Shine a penlight or cobalt blue light at an oblique angle across the cornea. Bright green areas indicate a true corneal abrasion. A minute corneal foreign body can be seen in the concentration of fluorescein in the area surrounding it.

    e. Irrigate eyes to prevent chemical conjunctivitis from the fluorescein.

  3. Evert the upper eyelid to examine the upper conjunctiva (Fig. 3-1):

    a. Instruct the patient to look down with both eyes.

    b. Grasp the eyelashes of the upper lid and gently pull the lid down and slightly outward away from the eye.

    c. Apply a gentle pressure directly on the lid (on the upper edge of the tarsus on the skin side, about 10 mm above the upper lid margin), using a small cotton-tipped applicator.

    d. Simultaneously pull the lashes upward.

    e. Examine the upper conjunctiva.

    f. Remove the foreign body if you see one (see Removal techniques).

    g. When the foreign body is removed release the upper lid and ask the patient to look up. The eye lid will readily flip back to its normal position.

4. Examine the lower eyelid:

    a. Have the patient fix his or her gaze upward, grasp the lower eyelashes, and pull the lid away from the eyeball.

    b. Place the tip of your free index finger on the cheek over the inferior orbital margin and push the skin upward to expose the lower lid conjunctiva.

5. Removal techniques:

    a. Instruct the patient to gaze on a distant object.

    b. Hold the eyelid apart with the thumb and index finger.

    c. Gently wipe the cornea or upper tarsal conjunctiva once with a sterile cotton swab moistened with sterile normal saline or ocular irrigating solution. If the particle does not dislodge with this gentle brushing maneuver, stop. The corneal epithelium could be damaged by continued swabbing.

    d. If the particle remains embedded, slip an eye spud or the beveled edge up of a 25-gauge needle attached to a syringe (some references recommend 18-gauge needle) under the particle and lift off the cornea. Several attempts may be necessary (Fig. 3-2, p. 104).

    e. Keep the instrument parallel to the surface of the cornea to prevent pressure, which could lead to perforation.

6. After the foreign body is removed, retest visual acuity and apply an antibiotic ointment and sterile eye pad.

Postprocedure patient education

Instruct the patient to return within 24 hours for reevaluation, and to call if there is any blurred vision. The majority of superficial injuries heal without difficulty.

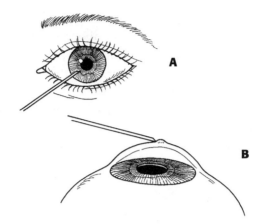

Fig. 3-2 **A** Removal of a superficial corneal foreign body. **B** Side view illustrates the thickness of the cornea relative to the beveled needle edge. The needle or eye spud should be tangential to the cornea, and the object should be gently scraped off the cornea. (From Pfenninger JL, Fowler GC: *Procedures for primary care physicians,* St Louis, 1994, Mosby.)

Warn the patient always to wash the hands with soap before applying an eye ointment, manipulating an eyelid, or touching any part of the eye.

Teach the patient how to instill an eye ointment: Pull down the lower lid and place a line of ointment just inside. Close the eye and look all around. Advise the patient that vision will be blurry after instillation; the patient should not attempt to drive or perform tasks that require hand-eye coordination.

For eye patches instruct the patient as follows: Keep the eye patch on for 24 hours. It is to rest the eye, so do not pull it off for even a short while. Vision will be affected, especially in the area of depth perception, so do not drive or perform tasks that require hand-eye coordination.

Advise the patient that it is best not to watch television or read while the patch is on or it may strain the other eye.

Instruct the patient to avoid rubbing the eyes.

Warn the patient that the foreign body sensation may return temporarily before patch removal when the anesthetic agent has worn off.

Tell the patient with contact lenses not to wear them until seen by an ophthalmologist.

Advise the patient to wear protective glasses when working around flying particles such as dust, sawdust, glass, metal, or sand.

Practitioner Followup/Complications

The anesthesia lasts about 15 minutes.

Corneal injuries usually heal within 24 hours after the foreign body is removed.

A followup examination by an ophthalmologist 1 to 2 days after the injury is recommended.

The patient should return to the ophthalmologist if symptoms are persistent or recurrent.

CPT BILLING CODE

65205—Removal of foreign body, external eye; conjunctival superficial.

BIBLIOGRAPHY

Clark RB, Farber JM, Sher NA: Eye emergencies and urgencies, *Patient Care* 15(1):24, 1989.

Driscoll CE: Removing a foreign body from the eye, *Patient Care* 30(5):145, 1988.

Holt GR, Holt JE: Management of orbital trauma and foreign bodies, *Otolaryngol Clin North Am,* 21(1):35, 1988.

Treatment of Corneal Abrasion

Description

Simple, minor corneal abrasions can be treated by the primary care provider. See the box for triage priority.

Indications

Treatment of corneal abrasion is warrented when there is any of the following:

- A history of the eye being scratched

Eye problems that need same-day care

Acute pain

Blurred vision that is not helped by repeated blinking or putting on glasses

Double vision

Pain involving contact lenses, especially extended-wear lenses

Seeing halos around objects (symptom of acute angle-closure glaucoma)

Seeing light flashes, black dots, or a curtain effect (symptom of retinal detachment)

Sensitivity to light, photophobia

Sudden loss of vision, with or without pain

Eye conditions that warrant immediate referral

Acute angle-closure glaucoma

Central retinal artery occlusion

Trauma to eye

Temporal arteritis

Vitreous hemorrhage

Retinal tear or detachment

Chemical burn (eye should be irrigated immediately then referred)

- Foreign body sensation and pain in eye
- Complaints of irritation in contact lens wearers (remove contact lens, evaluate, then refer to ophthalmologist)
- Photophobia (especially in children)

Contraindications/Precautions

Contact lens wearers should be referred to an ophthalmologist.

Practitioners avoid prescribing topical anesthetics. These products retard corneal healing and may allow corneal abrasion to progress to corneal ulcers.

Practitioners avoid prescribing steroids for the eye. They retard healing and promote overgrowth of virus and fungus.

Patient Preparation/Education

Tell the patients that they will not feel pain if anesthetic drops are used, but will feel pressure.

Equipment

- Snellen eye chart
- Sterile normal saline or ophthalmic irrigating solution
- Topical anesthetic drops (proparacaine HCl 0.5%)
- Topical antimicrobial ointment (sulfacetamide 10%)
- Fluorescein-impregnated strips
- Penlight or cobalt blue light
- Ophthalmoscope
- Eye patch and paper tape

Procedure

1. Obtain a history (full description of the current episode, past relevant history, allergies, etc.).
2. Check visual acuity.
3. If it is difficult for the patient to keep the eye open because of pain, instill 1 or 2 drops of topical anesthetic and wait about 1 minute.
4. Inspect the cornea and sclera using a light source. Open the lids wide using your thumb and index finger.
5. Apply fluorescein dye.
   a. Moisten the tip of the dye strip with sterile saline.
   b. Touch the strip to the conjunctiva. (If you are staining both eyes, use separate strips to prevent cross-contamination.)
   c. Instruct the patient to gently blink eye and look straight ahead.
   d. Shine the penlight or cobalt blue light at an oblique angle across the cornea. Bright green areas indicate a true corneal abrasion. A minute corneal foreign body can be seen in the concentration of fluorescein in the area surrounding it (Fig. 3-3, p. 108).

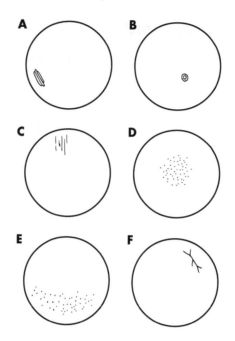

Fig. 3-3 Corneal defect staining patterns for specific injuries. **A** Typical abrasion. **B** Abrasion around a corneal foreign body. **C** Abrasion from a conjunctival foreign body under the upper lid. **D** Abrasion from excessive wearing of a contact lens. **E** Ultraviolet exposure (resulting from sunlamp exposure, welding, or snow blindness). **F** Herpetic dendritic keratitis. (From Pfenninger JL, Fowler GC: *Procedures for primary care physicians,* St Louis, 1994, Mosby.)

     e. Irrigate the eyes to prevent chemical conjunctivitis from the fluorescein.

6. If an abrasion is seen:
    a. Instill 1 or 2 drops of additional anesthetic.
    b. Instill a cycloplegic if the patient has significant spasm and pain (contraindicated in children).
    c. Apply an antibiotic ointment.
    d. Patch the eye firmly so the patient is unable to open it. Two patches may be needed (Fig. 3-4). Do not patch eyes in children under 1 year old.

7. Reexamine in 24 hours using fluorescein.
8. If the abrasion has healed, give antibiotic drops for 3 days.
9. If the abrasion is smaller, instill a cycloplegic and an antibiotic ointment, repatch, and examine again in 24 hours.

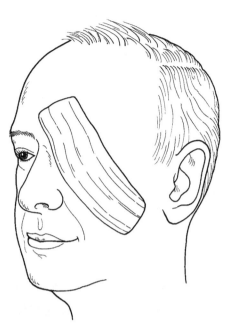

Fig. 3-4 Pressure eye patch. (From Pfenninger JL, Fowler GC: *Procedures for primary care physicians,* St Louis, 1994, Mosby.)

10. Refer to an ophthalmologist if the eye is not healing well, or if cloudiness or drainage appear.
11. Recheck visual acuity before discharging patient.

Postprocedure patient education

Instruct the patient to return in 24 hours for reevaluation.

The patient will need reevaluation every day until the abrasion is healed.

Advise the patient to keep eye patch on for 24 hours; to rest the eye; do not pull it off for even a short while.

Warn the patient not to drive or perform tasks that require hand-eye coordination because depth perception will be impaired by the patch.

Advise the patient that it is best not to watch television or read while the patch is on.

Practitioner Followup/Complications

Practitioners reevaluate the eye daily until the abrasion is healed. Practitioners refer to an ophthalmologist if the abrasion is not healing properly or signs and symptoms of infection occur.

Practitioners refer contact lens wearers to their ophthalmologists.

BIBLIOGRAPHY

Boyd-Monk H: Assessing acquired ocular diseases, *Nurs Clin North Am* 25(4):811, 1990.

Clark RB, Farber JM, Sher NA: Eye emergencies and urgencies, *Patient Care* Jan (1):24, 1989.

Elkington AR, Khaw PT: ABC of eyes. Injuries to the eye, *BMJ* 297(6641):122, 1988.

Hiatt RL: Eye trauma in children, *South Med J* 84(6):747, 1991.

Janda AM: Ocular trauma. Triage and treatment, *Postgrad Med* 90(7):51, 1991.

The Trouble with contact lenses, *Emergency Medicine,* 43, September 15, 1990.

Removal of a Foreign Body from the Ear

Description

It is not uncommon for a foreign object to become stuck in an ear canal. It is quite common for children, particularly toddlers, to put objects into their ear canals. Such objects as pebbles, beads, beans, folded paper, and button batteries are commonly found in children's ears. In adults, foreign bodies in the ear are usually objects (such as a match stick or cotton swab) that have been used to relieve itching or soreness in the ear. In all ages, the most common foreign bodies are insects that accidentally enter the ear canal. The main symptoms of a foreign body in the ear canal are sudden pain, a feeling of fullness, and noise in the ear (usually buzzing or roaring). Sometimes irritation of the nerves in the ear canal may cause hiccups. Children often do not complain of these symptoms but may have a discharge from the ear, especially if the object has been in the ear for some time.

Indications

Any foreign object lodged in the ear canal should be removed to prevent infection or disruption of tympanic membrane.

Contraindications/Precautions

Practitioners do not attempt the procedures if the patient has tympanostomy tubes.

Practitioners do not attempt foreign object removal with perforated, or recently perforated tympanic membranes.

Practitioners do not perform the procedure if there has been recent surgery on the middle ear.

Practitioners should use care if there is vegetable matter in the ear that may expand in the presence of water.

Patient Preparation/Education

Patients should be instructed that they may feel ear pressure while the instrument is within the ear canal and to alert the practitioner if pain occurs.

Equipment

The tools needed will vary depending on the foreign object and its location.

- Blunt ear curette or ear spoon
- Ear or 60-cc syringe
- Basin of warm water
- Emesis basin
- Towel
- Otoscope
- Chemical agent to kill insect (optional)—microscope oil, 2% lidocaine, 4% lidocaine, or 2% viscous lidocaine.

Procedure

Visualize the foreign object; if it is not immediately visible place the tip only of otoscope outside of ear canal and retract pinna superiorly and posteriorly to aid visualization (Fig. 3-5, p. 112).

1. If the object CANNOT be visualized, pour warm water into the

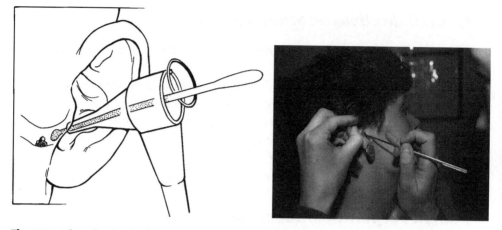

Fig. 3-5 Often, foreign bodies or cerumen in the ear canal can be removed under direct vision once careful, magnified otoscopic examination is completed. Notice how the patient's head is supported and the practitioner's hand rests on the face. (From Pfenninger JL, Fowler GC: *Procedures for primary care physicians,* St Louis, 1994, Mosby.)

clean basin; fill the irrigating syringe with warm water, expelling air; place the syringe tip into the canal; and direct a stream of water upward, not toward, the tympanic membrane. After irrigating the canal with 60 cc of water, examine the canal and the returned solution for the presence of the foreign object.

2. If the object CAN be visualized, retract the pinna superiorly and posteriorly with your nondominate hand, gently insert the curette or spoon along the canal until the object is grasped, and remove the object.

3. If a live insect is visualized, you should kill or immobilize it before you attempt to remove it. Place a chemical agent in the ear and wait for the insect to stop wiggling. Microscope oil kills the insects in about 45 seconds; lidocaine takes a bit longer.

Prescribe antibiotic ear drops if any injury has occurred to the canal.

Postprocedure patient education

Give the following instructions to patients or their caregivers:

Keep small objects out of reach of young children.
Tell children not to put objects into their ear but that if it happens again, to tell you or another adult immediately.

Notify the practitioner if there is any hearing loss or bleeding, continued pain, or discharge from the ear.

Practitioner Followup/Complications

The patient does not need to be seen for followup unless one of the following should occur:

- Bleeding
- Discharge
- Continuous ear pain
- Loss of hearing

CPT BILLING CODE

69200—Removal foreign body from external auditory canal without general anesthesia.

BIBLIOGRAPHY

Amundson L: Disorders of the external ear canal. In Vogt HB, editor: *Primary care, Disorders of the ears, nose, and throat*, Philadelphia, 1990, WB Saunders.

Capo JM, Lucente FE: Alkaline battery foreign bodies of the ear and nose, *Arch Otolaryngol Head Neck Surg* 112(5):562, 1986.

Frew M, Frew D: *Comprehensive medical assisting: administrative and clinical procedures*, Philadelphia, 1990, FA Davis.

Kavanagn KT, Litovitz T: Miniature battery foreign bodies in auditory and nasal cavities, *JAMA* 255(11):1470, 1986.

Leffler S, Cheney P, Tandberg D: Chemical immobilization and killing of intra-aural roaches, *Ann Emerg Med* 22(12):1795, 1993.

Rotello L: Removal of foreign bodies from the ear. In Jastremski MS, Dumas M, Penalver L, editors: *Emergency procedures*, Philadelphia, 1992, WB Saunders.

White SJ, Broner S: The use of acetone to dissolve a Styrofoam impaction of the ear, *Ann Emerg Med* 23(3):580, 1994.

Cerumen Disimpaction

Description

This is a procedure for removing cerumen from the ear canal.

Indications

This procedure may be necessary for visualization of the tympanic membrane to facilitate the diagnosis and treatment of otitis or other ear disease.

It may be needed for relief of dizziness, pressure sensation, or tinnitus.

It may be essential for enhancing auditory acuity if the ear is totally obstructed by cerumen.

A normal change of aging is decreased activity of the cerumen glands, causing reduced moisture. Dry cerumen is more likely to become impacted.

If an ear is obstructed and infection is not suspected, irrigation is warranted.

Contraindications/Precautions

If the purpose is to help visualize the tympanic membrane for signs of infection, do not irrigate. Instead, attempt to remove the wax plug with a cerumen spoon.

Practitioners do not attempt the procedure if there is suspected tympanic membrane perforation.

Practitioners do not perform it if the patient has a history of recent middle ear surgery.

Practitioners do not attempt it if the patient has tympanostomy tubes in place.

Practitioners do not perform this procedure if the patient has a history of multiple previous episodes of otitis media.

To avoid accidental tympanic membrane perforation, gentle pressure and irrigation should be used slowly.

The irrigating solution should be warm to prevent caloric stimulation.

The irrigating stream should be aimed at the superior wall of the ear canal instead of at the cerumen plug to avoid compaction of the plug against the tympanic membrane.

There is a potential for damage to the ear canal or tympanic membrane with an otoscope, cerumen spoon, or curette when a child is struggling.

Use of a papoose board or an immobilization device fashioned from sheets is less labor intensive and often safer than complete manual restraint.

In the older child, restraint may require one person assigned to each limb and a fifth to control the head.

Patient Preparation/Education

If possible, the patient should use wax softening ear drops for 3 to 5 days before the procedure.

Practitioners advise the patients that they may feel pressure, dizziness, or vertigo during the procedure.

The patients should alert the practitioner if pain or discomfort occurs.

The patient will need to assist with holding the basin.

Equipment

- Otoscope
- Irrigating apparatus: ear (or 60-cc) syringe, a pulsating water jet pump or a Water Pik on low setting. A regular syringe with a piece of 2-inch rubber tubing (e.g., from a sterile urinary catheter) on the end is adequate. The tubing from a butterfly needle is also adequate.
- Irrigating solution. Use a 1:1 mixture of warm water and hydrogen peroxide.
- Emesis basin
- Protective drapes, towels
- Cerumen spoon (optional)

Procedure

1. Position and drape the patient, preferably sitting upright. Have the patient hold the emesis basin under the ear. Put drapes on the patient's shoulder and neck (Fig. 3-6, p. 116).
2. Fill the syringe with body-temperature solution.
3. Retract the pinna posteriorly and superiorly with your nondomi-

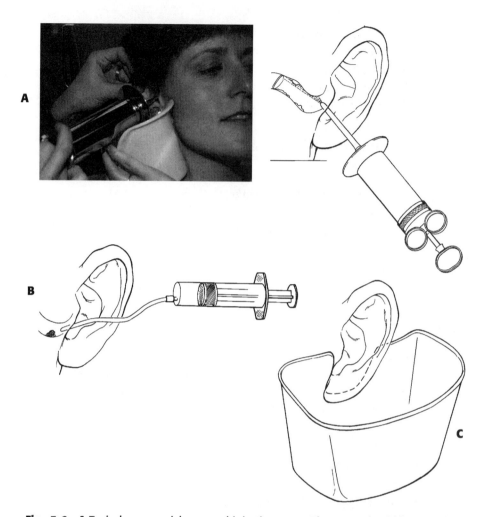

Fig. 3-6 **A** Typical commercial ear canal irrigation setup. The water should be at body temperature. The initial stream should be directed toward the superior canal. Patients often feel reassured when allowed to help hold the basin. Cover the upper torso with a splash bib. **B** Alternative irrigation setup. Butterfly tubing with needle and butterfly removed. **C** Basin cup that fits under ear. (From Pfenninger JL, Fowler GC: *Procedures for primary care physicians,* St Louis, 1994, Mosby.)

nant hand. (In a young child, pull down and forward.) Place the syringe tip at the canal opening without occluding the canal. Direct a gentle flow of solution toward the superior wall of the ear canal.

4. Irrigate each ear 2 or 3 times with full syringes, observing draining liquid for cerumen.
5. Inspect the ear. If wax remains, discontinue irrigation; send the

patient home to use liquid ear wax softener twice a day for 4 to 5 days and then return for repeat irrigation.

6. Discontinue the procedure if the patient complains of discomfort, as a precaution against an unrecognized perforation.
7. Inspect the canal after the procedure to ensure that there is no remaining wax.

Postprocedure patient education

Consider having the patient mix 50% rubbing alcohol and 50% white vinegar and apply drops of it once a day after bathing to the ear canal for 2 to 3 days after the procedure to prevent otitis externa.

Instruct the patient to call or return if any of following symptoms occur: hearing loss, ear pain or fullness, discharge, tinnitus.

Emphasize that cerumen is normal and is secreted by outer ear glands to protect the ear from bacteria.

If the patient works around flour, hay, dust, or other particles, debris may become caught and dried in the ear wax.

Some people, especially the elderly, may require regular ear hygiene. Advise the patient to use 2 drops of baby or mineral oil once or twice a week to soften wax so that it expels itself, or to purchase wax softening ear drops and use as directed on package.

Remind the patient it is important never to put anything in ear canal, especially commercial cotton tip applicators.

Practitioner Followup/Complications

No followup is necessary unless the patient experiences symptoms.

Unnecessary excess force may result in perforation of the tympanic membrane with possible loss of hearing.

Minor canal wall abrasions or otitis externa may follow overzealous irrigation or irrigation of extremely dry, hard wax.

Tinnitus may be produced by cold stimulation of the vestibular system.

CPT BILLING CODE

69210—Removal impacted cerumen (separate procedure), one or both ears.

BIBLIOGRAPHY

Macknin ML, Talo H, Medendrop SV: Effect of cotton-tipped swab use on ear-wax occlusion, *Clin Pediatr* 33(1):14, 1994.

Sharp J: Ear wax removal in general practice, *Nurs Times,* 87(19):45, 1991.

Sharp JF, and others: Ear wax removal: a survey of current practice, *BMJ* 301(6763): 1251, 1990.

Zivic R, King S: Cerumen-impaction management for clients of all ages, *Nurse Practitioner* 18(3):32, 1993.

Ear Piercing

Description

This procedure entails aseptically piercing the earlobes for cosmetic reasons. This is a procedure that primary care practitioners may periodically be asked to perform. There are two methods by which the earlobe can be pierced. The first method uses a disposable sterile needle; the second uses some sort of device or instrument. Ear piercing "guns" are available from several manufacturers and all operate using the same principles. The spring action on the "gun" forces either an earring or a surgical steel stud through the lobe. Because of the risk to practitioners of accidentally piercing their own skin with the needle, the "gun" method is safer and is described in this procedure.

There are a variety of devices for ear piercing. Some are similar to staple guns. For example, ERI Laboratories of Van Nuys, California, makes a "gun" that features a surgical steel stud that pierces the earlobe. It is of benefit to individuals who have an allergy to nickel, which is commonly found in costume jewelry and gold jewelry that is less than 24 karat. Inverness Corporation of Fairlawn, New Jersey, makes a "gun" that utilizes presterilized capsules containing earrings, which are inserted into the gun. The benefit is that the instrument does not come into contact with the ear. Nemsco of Norwen, Massachusetts, makes the Coren PS disposable earpiercer. The earring is imbedded in a plastic case that is pressed firmly to release the earring and shoot it through the earlobe.

Indications

The procedure is requested by the patient or a child (with parental permission).

Contraindications/Precautions

Practitioners do not use the procedure if there is an epidermoid cyst or local skin infection.

The procedure is contraindicated with a history of keloid formation.

Do not pierce ears if the patient has an immunodeficiency or coagulation disorder.

Individuals who are allergic to nickel (approximately 10% to 20% of the population) can develop a contact dermatitis to earrings after the ears have been pierced. It is manifested as a pruritic, erythematous rash on the lobes. A patch test can be done to confirm this allergy. Individuals with a nickel allergy should be instructed to wear earrings made of surgical stainless steel or 24 karat gold.

Piercing the helix should be discouraged. The blood supply of the helix is limited. This results in longer healing and increased susceptibility to infection.

Patient Preparation/Education

Practitioners instruct patients that they will feel a quick pinch or pressure as the lobe is pierced.

If the patients desire, ice cubes or topical anesthetic may be used before the procedure to anesthetize the ear lobe. Practitioners may have the patients hold the earlobe between two ice cubes for 1 to 2 minutes.

Equipment

- Ear-piercing kit (gun, needles, and backing)
- Surgical skin-marking pencil or marker
- 70% isopropyl alcohol swabs or povidone–iodine solution (Betadine)

- Ice cubes or topical anesthetic (optional)

Procedure

1. Position the patient on a stool or elevate the exam table so that the ears are at practitioner's eye level.
2. Clean the earlobe, front and back, with an alcohol swab.
3. Anesthetize the earlobe or squeeze it between your thumb and index finger for about 30 seconds.
4. Use a surgical marking pen to place a small dot on the earlobe where the ear is to be pierced (Fig. 3-7). This ensures correct placement. Do not place the dot too low or heavy earrings may cause the hole to tear out. For the first ear piercing, place the dot on the center of each earlobe. For a second ear piercing, have the patient remove existing earrings. Following the natural line of the earlobe, place the dot approximately ⅜ inch up from the first hole. For the third ear piercing, have the patient remove existing earrings. Following the natural line of the earlobe, place the dot approximately ⅜ inch up from the second hole. Have the patient check the position of the dots in a mirror. If the patient is dissatisfied, remove the dots using an alcohol swab and mark again.

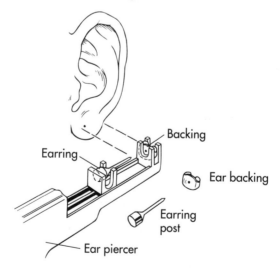

Fig. 3-7 Ear-piercing technique.

5. Position the earlobe between the front and rear portions of the piercing device; the nose of the device should be over the placement dot.
6. Gently squeeze the handle of the piercing device until the earring has been released from the device and has been inserted in the earring back. The earlobe is now pierced.
7. Release your hand pressure on the device and gently pull the earlobe forward to free the earring back.
8. Repeat the process for the other ear.
9. If the ear is pierced in the wrong location, remove the earring and apply pressure to the site. Do not repierce for at least 24 hours.

Postprocedure patient education

Give the patient the following instructions:
Avoid strong soaps, cosmetics, and hair spray on the newly pierced earlobes.

Keep hands and hair away from the newly pierced earlobe.

Wash hands with soap and water before touching the ear. Use a cotton swab moistened with alcohol to clean the earlobe twice a day.

Rotate the earrings twice a day to prevent crusting.

If the earlobe begins to get dry or flaky, stop using alcohol; instead, use an antibacterial ointment such as Bacitracin twice a day.

If the earlobe becomes tender, red, and crusty, apply hot compresses and then bacitracin ointment two to three times a day. If this continues for longer than three days call the practitioner. The earrings may need to be removed so the area can heal.

The studs or earrings must remain in place for 6 weeks before being removed or replaced with different earrings. This allows complete healing and epithelialization of the earlobe sinus tract.

Practitioner Followup/Complications

Practitioners watch for the development of local infection, cyst formation, or sepsis.

Practitioners evaluate for keloid formation.

Practitioners check for earlobe deformity with earring tearing through the skin.

Practitioners may find an embedded earring stud or backing if the patient has the backing on too tightly.

CPT BILLING CODE

69090—Ear piercing.

BIBLIOGRAPHY

George J, White M: Infections as a consequence of ear piercing, *Practitioner,* 233, 1989.

Graber R: Procedures for your practice, *Patient Care,* 194-196, 1990.

Epistaxis and Nasal Packing

Description

This procedure uses cauterization and packing of the nose to control nasal bleeding that has not resolved with direct pressure. In up to 90% of cases, epistaxis originates in the anterior septum in the rich vascular plexus known as Kisselbach's plexus or Little's area. Kisselbach's plexus is composed of the terminal septal branches of the anterior and posterior ethmoid arteries, the superior labial artery (via the external facial artery), and the sphenopalatine artery. Epistaxis may occur because of spontaneous rupture of vessels in the anterior nasal septum (mainly in children or the elderly); drying of the nares, which results in mucosal cracking; direct trauma; picking of the nostrils; hypertension (rarely); and blood dyscrasia.

Most childhood nosebleeds occur before age 10 and are anterior in location, usually from Little's area. Posterior bleeds are unusual in children and are signaled by inability to identify the bleeding site and continued oozing of blood into the pharynx despite treatment.

Trauma is the most frequent cause of nosebleeds in children. The patient's own finger is the most common source. Repeated local trauma causes an inflammatory response, and subsequent granulation tissue can be "picked off," causing bleeding. Nasal foreign bodies can traumatize the nasal mucosa as well.

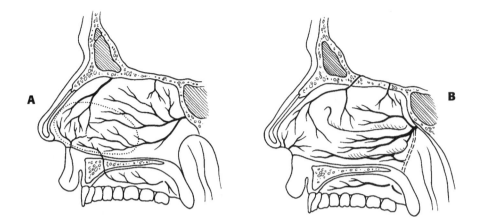

Fig. 3-8 A Blood supply to the nasal septum. Little's or Kiesselbach's area, the most common site of epistaxis, is delineated by a dotted line. **B** Blood supply to lateral nasal wall. Familiarity with blood supply as it relates to anatomy of the nose greatly enhances the practitioner's ability to control nasal bleeding.

Breathing dry air is a major predisposing factor to nosebleeds. Additionally, a deviated nasal septum may cause the nasal cavity on one side to be relatively narrowed; air passes through the narrowed side at a greater velocity, predisposing that side to nosebleeds.

Repeated infection and allergic rhinitis in childhood are also associated with nosebleeds. Repeated forceful nose blowing can rupture the septal venous vessels. Viral or bacterial rhinitis are also associated with increased vascularity of the inflamed nasal septum.

Indications

This procedure is performed to control nasal hemorrhage that has not been alleviated with firm pressure.

Contraindications/Precautions

Practitioners should use these procedures carefully if granulocytopenia is present. The relative severity of the hemorrhage needs to be weighed against the risk of life-threatening infection.

Practitioners do not attempt these procedures with known or suspected cribriform fracture or necrosis of the septum.

Severe epistaxis is not a simple event. The practitioner should have the proper equipment readily available in case the patient has syncope or goes into shock, cardiac arrest, or pulmonary distress. Epinephrine and ephedrine should be used with caution or not at all in patients with severe hypertension. Unless shock is present, epistaxis should not be treated with the patient in a supine position.

The partial pressure of oxygen in the blood often decreases 10 mm mercury from the packing in the nose as the result of nasopulmonary reflexes. This decrease, in conjunction with hypovolemia, hypertension, and preexisting pulmonary disease, can precipitate a stroke or a myocardial infarction in susceptible individuals. Therefore an electrocardiogram should be obtained in patients more than 40 years old, and referral for workup should be performed in patients with pulmonary, renal, or cardiac disease.

Posterior bleeding is unusual in children and is suspected when a bleeding site cannot be visualized and an anterior pack fails to control the bleeding. Posterior bleeding should be managed by an otolaryngologist in the hospital, where ligation or embolization of the vessel may be performed. Additionally, if bilateral anterior packs are indicated the patient will need to be referred to an otolaryngologist for possible hospital admission.

Patient Preparation/Education

The patient or the practitioner should maintain constant pressure on the nose by pinching it between the thumb and first finger as close to the facial bones as possible (Fig. 3-9).

The practitioners must provide reassurance to the patient throughout the entire procedure, making sure to explain each step to the patient before carrying out the packing.

Also, the patient needs to be made aware that nosebleeds, although messy and upsetting, are rarely life threatening.

Practitioners make sure the patient knows that bleeding will be controlled at the end of the procedure.

It is important to explain that the nostril will feel full and will not be easy to breathe through.

It is also important to explain that some pressure may be felt during cauterization but that pain should not be felt if the mucosa is properly anesthetized.

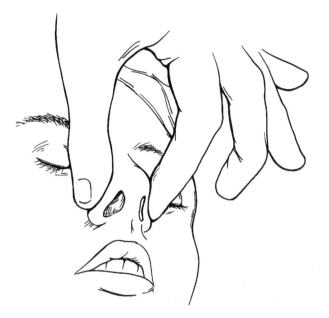

Fig. 3-9 Apply pressure by pinching the nose to stop the bleeding. (From Pfenninger JL, Fowler GC: *Procedures for primary care physicians,* St Louis, 1994, Mosby.)

Practitioners ask questions to determine the patient's general physical condition, amount of blood lost, and the possibility of a coagulopathy. Previous bleeding episodes and methods of control should be explored. A history of trauma, surgery, allergy, recent upper respiratory infection, or a foreign body should be elicited.

Practitioners note the patient's vital signs. Orthostatic hypotension is an important clue to moderate to severe volume loss. In children, an increase in heart rate of 10% to 15% is indicative of significant volume loss.

Practitioners inspect the patient for signs of hemorrhagic disease (e.g., ecchymoses, petechiae, organomegaly, telangiectasia).

Equipment

- Light source, preferably head lamp
- Nasal speculum
- Suction apparatus, including Fraser tips No. 5 to No. 8, 8-10 French suction catheter
- Cautery unit or silver nitrate sticks (optional)

- Topical thrombin or other topical coagulant (optional)
- Topical vasoconstrictor such as epinephrine 1:1000 or phenylephrine 0.125% to 0.5%
- Expandable nasal sponges or petrolatum gauze packing
- Bayonet forceps
- Kidney basin

Procedure

Attempt cauterization of the bleeding site, if visualized, first. If the site is unsuitable for cauterization, or if cauterization fails to control the bleeding, perform tamponade of the bleeding area with gauze.

1. Identify the specific site of bleeding. This is the key to success.
2. The patient should be seated, leaning forward, in a "sniffing position."
3. Before the examination have the patient blow his or her nose to clear the nasal passages of blood clots. Suction will serve the same purpose in an uncooperative child.
4. Following the removal of clots and blood, place the nasal speculum into the nares and inspect the nasal cavity for a bleeding source. Begin with the nares from which the blood first originated. Inspect the nasal cavity from anterior to posterior. Use the head lamp for better visualization.
5. To control bleeding if pressure is not successful, try packing the nose with topical thrombin, followed by 10 minutes of firm and constant pressure, by squeezing the anterior cartilage of the nose between the thumb and index finger. This technique is safer and technically simpler than using silver nitrate sticks.
6. If the bleeding is still not controlled, topical application of a vasoconstrictor, such as neosynephrine, or epinephrine with a cotton pledget for 5 to 10 minutes is often effective. CAUTION: Although only minimal volumes of these drugs are necessary, care should be taken to anticipate and treat any untoward effects from systemic absorption.
7. If you decide to cauterize, use silver nitrate sticks to touch the area around the bleeding site for 5 to 10 minutes. Work in concentric circles, starting away from the bleeding site. The mucosa may

turn gray to black. Note: you cannot cauterize an actively bleeding site with silver nitrate. More vasoconstrictor may be required to stop the bleeding.
8. If bleeding persists, proceed with nasal packing. Nasal sponges are now available for this purpose. They are inserted dry and expand when wet. They can be cut to fit any child. Also petroleum gauze packing may be used.
9. Insert the packing into the nose:
    a. Hold the nasal speculum in your nondominant hand and use your dominant hand to manipulate the bayonet forceps.
    b. Grasp the gauze strip with the bayonet forces, forming a loop that leaves the end of the packing outside the nose (Fig. 3-10, *A*, p. 128).
    c. Pack the anterior nasal cavity from top to bottom by inserting successive loops of packing into the nose. Each loop should be placed under the previous loops in an accordion fashion and as far posterior as possible (Fig. 3-10, *B*).
    d. Fill the nostril, but not too tightly because excessive pressure may cause ischemic necrosis.
    e. When the nostril is fully packed, secure both ends of the nasal pack to the external cheek to prevent the ends from falling into the nasopharynx.
    f. Packing can be removed in 2 to 4 days.

Postprocedure patient education

Give the patient the following instructions:

- Use no aspirin or nonsteroidal antiinflammatory medications for the next 3 to 4 days.
- You may take a decongestant or antihistamine for excessive mucus production.
- Do not blow your nose with the packing in your nostrils.
- Apply petroleum jelly to the nares daily for 4 to 5 days.
- Avoid strenuous physical activity, bending, and sneezing if possible.
- Follow up with the health provider if nosebleeds persist.
- Place nothing in the nostrils.
- Run a humidifier in the house during winter months, especially at night.

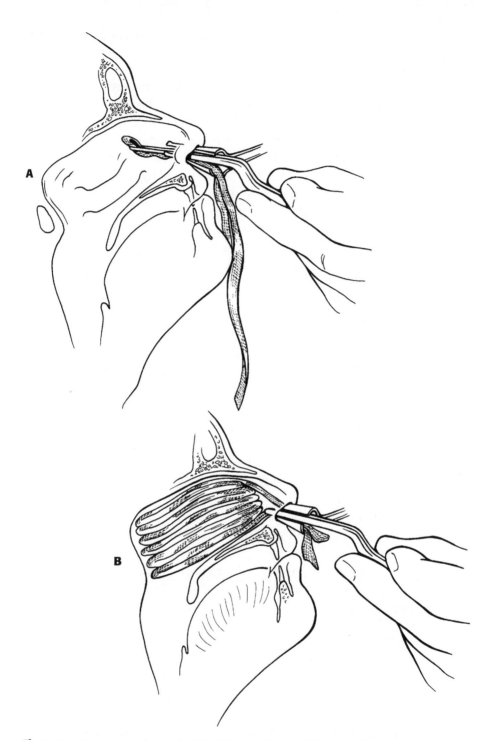

Fig. 3-10 **A** Insert anterior pack with folded end inserted first. **B** Fold gauze pack in layers. (From Pfenninger JL, Fowler GC: *Procedures for primary care physicians,* St Louis, 1994, Mosby.)

- Avoid alcohol. Alcohol can also increase the risk of rebleeding.
- If bleeding recurs, apply pressure for 10 minutes while compressing the soft and bony parts of the nose.
- Call the practitioner when there is development of unexplained bruises; if bleeding recurs and cannot be controlled by pressure, or when there is respiratory distress, airway obstruction, or fever.

Teach parents and the child, if he or she is old enough, the signs and symptoms of infection.

Teach parents and the child, if he or she is old enough, the signs and symptoms of respiratory distress and airway obstruction.

Packing should be removed only by a health care provider.

Practitioner Followup/Complications

Practitioners arrange for the patient to be seen in 24 to 48 hours for removal of the packing.

Antibiotic coverage should be provided while the packing·is in place. The drug of choice is usually amoxicillin. Alternatives are erythromycin or Augmentin.

Decongestants may be prescribed while the packing is in place.

Tylenol or tylenol with codeine should be prescribed depending on the degree of discomfort.

Practitioners must be alert for the development of:

- Syncope during packing
- Local infection
- Sinusitis
- Toxic shock syndrome
- Bacteremia
- Iatrogenic sleep apnea
- Airway obstruction secondary to displacement of packing into nasopharynx

CPT BILLING CODE

30901—Control nasal hemorrhage, anterior, simple (limited cautery and/or packing) any method.

30903—Control nasal hemorrhage, anterior, complex (extensive cautery and/or packing) any method.

BIBLIOGRAPHY

Halloran TH: Nasal packing: stopping excessive blood loss, *Nursing* 23(10):32, 1993.

Jastremski M: *Emergency procedures,* Philadelphia, 1992, WB Saunders.

Josephson GD, Godley FA, Stierna P: Practical management of epistaxis, *Med Clin North Am* 75(6):1311, 1991.

Petruzzelli GJ, Johnson JT: How to stop a nosebleed, *Postgrad Med* 86(4):44, 1989.

Reisdorff E, Roberts M, Wiegenstein J: *Pediatric emergency medicine,* Philadelphia, 1993, WB Saunders.

Toner JG, Walby AP: Comparison of electro and chemical cautery in the treatment of anterior epistaxis, *J Laryngol Otol* 104(8):617, 1990.

Removal of a Foreign Body from the Nose

Description

This procedure describes the use of appropriate instrumentation to extricate a foreign body that is positioned forward of the pharynx and can be visualized with a speculum.

The extent of tissue reaction and bleeding that ensues is largely a function of the size, position, movement, and antigenicity of the foreign body. The only limits on the size and shape of nasal foreign bodies are the physical limits of the cavities into which they are placed.

Foreign bodies can remain unnoticed for long periods of time. A rhinolith is a nasal foreign body that has become mineralized. A rhinolith will continue to increase in size as mineral salts are deposited onto its surface. It is usually an incidental finding on plain x-ray radiogram.

Retained foreign bodies can be classified as animal, vegetable, or mineral. The primary reason for making these distinctions is the somewhat different approaches to their removal. Insects and other animate objects should be killed before removal is attempted. Vegetable matter tends to swell if moistened and should be removed in a dry environment if possible. Foreign objects that are round and plastic can be difficult to grasp.

Vasoconstriction enlarges the nostril slightly, thereby easing the movement of the foreign body, and also minimizes bleeding. In a very young or uncooperative patient, sedation may be appropriate to minimize trauma and prevent aspiration.

Foreign bodies that are most commonly found in children's noses include such objects as buttons, beads, cotton, beans, and other objects of appropriate size. Vegetable foreign bodies will absorb water from the nasal mucosa and swell with time, making removal much more difficult than insertion.

Indications

A child or adult with a retained nasal foreign body often presents with a foul odor from the nostrils, unilateral purulent rhinorrhea, or persistent epistaxis. More commonly, the patient presents with the request for object removal.

Contraindications/Precautions

The practitioner should not attempt to remove foreign bodies not easily visualized or requiring general anesthesia to remove.

If a foreign body is large and initial attempts to remove it are unsuccessful, the procedure is likely to cause trauma or aspiration and referral to an otolaryngologist is indicated.

Practitioners should not push the object further into the nasopharynx, hoping that the object will be swallowed, because aspiration may occur.

Practitioners do not irrigate, because the nasal cavity is open posteriorly and aspiration may occur.

If it appears that prolonged attempts at removal are required, refer the patient to a specialist.

The very young or uncooperative patient may require sedation to prevent trauma during extraction.

It is important to examine both nares and ears carefully even when only a single foreign body is suspected. It is not uncommon for children to place objects in both their nose and their ears.

Patient Preparation/Education

Provide reassurance throughout the entire procedure, explaining each step as it is performed.

It is important for the patient to remain still, so as to minimize trauma to the nasal passage during the procedure.

Advise the patient that the nostril may feel full or numb from the topical anesthesia.

Equipment

- Headlight or head mirror
- Nasal speculum (Fig. 3-11)
- Topical anesthetic (4% lidocaine) and vasoconstrictor (0.25% phenylephrine HCl)
- Immobilization device (optional)
- One of the following depending on the foreign body:
  Suction and several suction tips (8 to 10 French cath)
  Alligator or Hartmann forceps
  Wire loop or curette
  Bayonet forceps
  Right angle hooks
  No. 4 Fogarty catheter

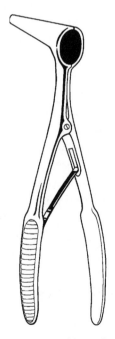

Fig. 3-11   Nasal speculum.

Procedure

1. Try to determine type of object in the nostril by history from the patient or the parent to determine the best approach to removal.
2. Position the patient erect, sitting, with the head tilted forward (more of the nasal cavity is visible in this position than with the head tilted back).
3. Use the nasal speculum to visualize the nostril.
4. Apply a topical anesthetic or vasoconstrictor as spray or drops. If tissue edema is present in the nares, the practitioner can ease the removal of the foreign body by applying a topical vasoconstrictor.
5. In cooperative children, occlude the unobstructed nostril, keep the mouth closed, and have the children forcefully blow their nose. This may be attempted up to 15 times.
6. Determine which instrument provides the best chance for removing of the foreign body. Choice of instrument for removal of a foreign body is largely related to its exact location, shape, and composition and the practitioner's preference.

   - Smooth, round objects can be removed with suction or with right-angle hooks.
   - A bayonet forceps can be used to grasp an object with a small leading edge (Fig. 3-12, p. 134).
   - Objects that may break when grasped may be more easily removed with a curette or wire loop (Fig. 3-13, p. 135).
   - A No. 4 Fogarty vascular catheter may be used to remove blunt nasal foreign bodies in children. Pass the catheter beyond the foreign body and inflate the balloon. Maintain slow gentle traction on the catheter while carefully extricating the object. This technique may be less traumatic than removal with a forceps.
   - In some cases, a lubricated No. 8 Foley catheter may be passed beneath and beyond the object, inflated with 2 to 3 ml of water, and slowly withdrawn.
   - The Fogarty catheter may also be used to stabilize the foreign body from behind while it is removed with forceps, because

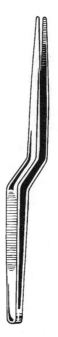

Fig. 3-12   Bayonet forceps.

attempts to remove a foreign body may otherwise result in the object being forced into the oral pharynx.

Postprocedure patient education

After extraction, any intranasal bleeding can be tamponaded with a small pack of gauze moistened with 0.5% phenylephrine.

Residual inflammation of the nasal membranes should clear spontaneously in a few days.

Instruct the patient to follow up with the provider if prolonged bleeding occurs.

Teach patients or their parents the signs and symptoms of sinus infection and otitis media.

Talk to parents of young children about how to:

- Child-proof their house.
- Remove small objects within children's reach.
- Provide careful supervision of young children.
- Understand normal growth and development: hand to mouth ac-

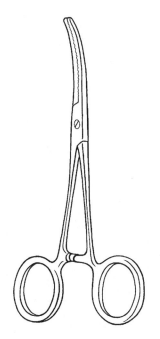

Fig. 3-13 Curved forceps hemostat.

tivity, children's natural curiosity to stick objects in orifices (nose, mouth, ears).

Practitioner Followup/Complications

Use care during this procedure to prevent posterior dislodging of the object because the patient may swallow or aspirate it.

Aspiration of the object into the tracheobronchial tree may precipitate bronchospasm, as manifested by shortness of breath and wheezing. This requires referral to an emergency room for bronchoscopic removal under anesthesia.

Instruct the patient or parents in the management of epistaxis, which may occur if nasal tissue has been irritated during foreign body removal.

Complications can occur as a result of the foreign body itself, the examination, or the removal.

Infection can closely follow the presence of a foreign body. The sinus ostia in the anterior section of the nose and eustachian tube in the posterior section of the nose can become blocked, predisposing the patient to sinusitis or otitis media. Signs of infection should be treated.

If an object is not removed in a timely manner, a rhinolith may form. Its size gradually increases and may complicate removal or predispose the patient to serious infection.

CPT BILLING CODE

30300—Removal foreign body, intranasal; office type procedure.

BIBLIOGRAPHY

Capo JM, Lucente FE: Alkaline battery foreign bodies of the ear and nose, *Arch Otolaryngol Head Neck Surg* 112(5):562, 1986.

Kavanagh KT, Litovitz T: Miniature battery foreign bodies in auditory and nasal cavities, *JAMA* 255(11):1470, 1986.

Nandapalan V, McIlwain JC: Removal of nasal foreign bodies with a Fogarty biliary balloon catheter, *J Laryngol Otol* 108(9):758, 1994.

Templer J: Removing foreign bodies from the nose, *Hosp Med* 8:35, 1990.

CHAPTER 4

Respiratory Procedures

Nebulizer Treatment

Description

This procedure is required for the delivery of drugs via aerosolization. These drugs may loosen and mobilize pulmonary secretions, promote clearance of secretions by liquification, and enhance airway exchange through bronchodilation.

Indications

Use nebulizers to aid in the treatment of moderate asthma or reactive airway disease in ambulatory outpatients.

Use this procedure as an adjunct in the management of symptoms resulting from COPD or other processes compromising the respiratory system.

Contraindications/Precautions

Practitioners do not use a nebulizer if the patient is unable to take deep breaths, because precise dosing cannot be achieved.

Practitioners do not use a nebulizer if the patient cannot tolerate aerosol because of nausea, vomiting, "shakiness," or tachycardia.

Patient Preparation/Education

Practitioners instruct the patients to sit up as straight as possible for maximum chest expansion.

Practitioners instruct the patients to inhale normally during the treatment and, after every third breath, to inhale deeply holding their breath for two counts before exhaling.

Equipment

- Air compressor unit nebulizer
- Mouthpiece
- Flex tube
- Manifold with medicine cup
- Connecting tubing
- Stethoscope
- Medication

Procedure

1. Place the medication in the medicine cup.
2. Perform a chest assessment of the patients and check pulse if a sympathomimetic drug is to be administered.
3. Have the patients hold the nebulizer upright and close their lips around the mouthpiece. With young children, use the mask attachment over the nose and mouth.
4. Have the patients breathe into the machine until the medication is gone.
5. When the therapy is complete, check the patients' pulse, auscultate their chest, and observe for effectiveness or side effects.
6. Disassemble the equipment, rinse it with a germicidal solution, rinse it with water and dry it completely. In some cases the equipment used is disposable.

Postprocedure patient education

Encourage the patients to cough following the procedure in order to dislodge loosened secretions.

The patients may rinse their mouth if the aerosol leaves a bad taste.

Practitioner Followup/Complications

The practitioner should observe for complications of the particular medication used.

BIBLIOGRAPHY

Erl B, Robbins P: Hand-held nebulizer therapy, *J Pediatr Nurs* 5(6):408, 1990.

Hung JC, Hambleton G, Super M: Evaluation of two commercial jet nebulisers and three compressors for the nebulisation of antibiotics, *Arch Dis Child* 71(4):335, 1994.

Idris AH and others: Emergency department treatment of severe asthma. Metered-dose inhaler plus holding chamber is equivalent in effectiveness to nebulizer, *Chest* 103(3):661, 1993.

Kerem E and others: Efficacy of albuterol administered by nebulizer versus spacer device in children with acute asthma, *J Pediatr Aug* 123(2):313, 1993.

Nathan RA and others: Multicenter dose-ranging study of bitolterol mesylate solution for nebulization in children with asthma, *Ann Allergy* 72(3):209, 1994.

Singh M, Kumar L: Continuous nebulised salbutamol and oral once a day prednisolone in status asthmaticus, *Arch Dis Child* 69(4):416, 1993.

Spirometry

Description

This procedure is utilized to measure airflow into and out of the lungs for the purpose of diagnosing pulmonary disease. The rate of airflow from the lungs during a spirometric test is determined by the elastic recoil of the lungs and the patency of the pulmonary airways as well as the condition of the respiratory muscles and/or the patient's muscular effort. Lungs have a tendency to collapse because they are elastic and under pressure from the thoracic cage.

Opposed to this tendency to collapse is the airway resistance. If airway resistance is high (bronchospasm, edema, mucus plugs, inflammation), airflow from the lungs is limited and air trapping occurs. This happens in obstructive disease such as chronic obstructive pulmonary disease (COPD), asthma, and emphysema. In restrictive disease, the lungs lose their elastic capabilities because of fibrosis. They are not able to inflate adequately, so lung volumes are low. The rate of airflow, however, does not drop until restriction is severe or if obstructive defects coexist. This commonly occurs in sarcoidosis and asbestosis.

Indications

This test may be a part of a standard workup of dyspnea, chronic cough, chest tightness, or cough with exercise.

Spirometry is used in the evaluation of smokers over the age of 40.

This test indicates residual damage to the lungs from occupational exposure to dust and chemicals.

Spirometry may be part of presurgical testing for some patients.

Spirometry is often used to evaluate the adequacy of management of patients on bronchodilators.

Spirometry is used in the documentation of pulmonary disability.

This test is used in screening of patients with systemic disease that can involve the lungs, such as rheumatoid arthritis, systemic lupus erythematosus, or sarcoidosis.

Contraindications/Precautions

Practitioners do not attempt Spirometry in the presence of severe shortness of breath, severe fatigue, or if the patient is uncooperative.

Patient Preparation/Education

Practitioners explain that this procedure is painless and that all the patient has to do is breathe into the device.

If the patients are obese, the practitioner can have them stand; other patients should sit.

Nose clips are recommended.

The practitioner should have the patient remove any dentures and restrictive clothing.

The practitioner demonstrates the maneuvers. The procedure should be explained and demonstrated even if the patient has done the test before. The practitioner can explain to the patient that the machine measures how much and how fast air leaves the lungs. Before the demonstration, say, "You need to take a deep breath, as much as you possibly can, until you can't hold anymore. Like this." The practitioner demonstrates how the mouthpiece is placed in the mouth, with the teeth around the outside, and lips closed tightly around it. Then the practitioner instructs the patient to "Blow out as hard and as fast as possible, try to force all the air you can from your lungs." The practitioner may show how to blow through the mouthpiece using body language to emphasize the importance of maximal inhalation, maximal force, and a prolonged effort. The practitioner emphasizes how to squeeze the last little bit of air out of the lungs for the most accurate result.

The practitioner asks if they have any questions.

Procedure

1. Gather patient information—name, age, sex, height without shoes, weight, race, and a short respiratory history.
2. Calibrate the machine. Follow the instructions for your machine.
3. Put a new mouthpiece on the spirometer and have the patient try it. Encourage the patient to relax. Prompt inhalation with, "Now take a deep breath." Coax the patient with "MORE, MORE, ALL YOU CAN HOLD." Make sure there is a tight seal on the mouthpiece. Then prompt exhalation with "NOW BLAST IT OUT HARD AND FAST!! ALL YOU CAN. MORE. MORE. KEEP ON GOING!" You must coax for at least 6 seconds and as much as 10 seconds.
4. Repeat the procedure. There should be at least three acceptable maneuvers. The American Thoracic Society defines an acceptable and reproducible spirogram as having the two largest forced vital capacity (FVC) measurements within 5% of each other and

the two largest 1-second forced expiratory volume (FEV1) must match within 5%.

5. To evaluate for reversibility, administer a beta-agonist with a bronchodilator via a hand-held inhaler.
6. Wait about 20 minutes and then repeat the above procedure.

Interpretation of results

DEFINITIONS NEEDED TO UNDERSTAND SPIROMETRY

- Tidal volume (TV)—Normal flow of air in a resting subject; normal is 500 ml.
- Inspiratory reserve volume (IRV)—Additional amount of air inhaled over and above the tidal volume; normal is 3 L.
- Expiratory reserve volume (ERV)—Volume of air exhaled from the resting position; normal is 1.1 L.
- Forced vital capacity (FVC)—Sum of TV, ERV, and IRV, or the total amount one can exhale after taking the deepest breath; normal is 3.88 to 5.0 L.
- Forced expiratory volume in one second (FEV1)—The volume of the FVC is exhaled in one second; normal is 3.12 to 3.96 L.
- Percentage of FEV1—Volume of the FVC (FEV1/FVC); normal is 65% to 85%

INTERPRETATION OF SPIROMETRY MADE EASY

Typical spirograms are shown in Figure 4-1.

The degree of obstruction = Reduced maximal expiratory flow = Reduced FEV1 and % FEV1.

The degree of restriction = Reduced volume = Reduced FVC (normal % FEV1)

The FEV1/FVC ratio detects early obstruction. Since FVC decreases with increasing obstruction, it is not useful in advanced disease.

Reduction of the FVC and %FEV1 may have one of two causes:

1. Obstructive and restrictive disease.
2. The FVC is low because of chronic airway obstruction. If the FVC gets better following bronchodilator then the patient has chronic obstruction.

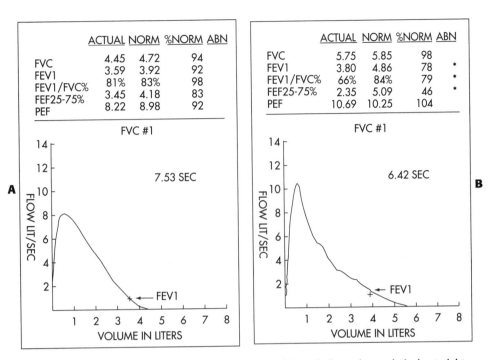

	ACTUAL	NORM	%NORM	ABN
FVC	4.45	4.72	94	
FEV1	3.59	3.92	92	
FEV1/FVC%	81%	83%	98	
FEF25-75%	3.45	4.18	83	
PEF	8.22	8.98	92	

	ACTUAL	NORM	%NORM	ABN
FVC	5.75	5.85	98	
FEV1	3.80	4.86	78	*
FEV1/FVC%	66%	84%	79	*
FEF25-75%	2.35	5.09	46	*
PEF	10.69	10.25	104	

Fig. 4-1 A Normal spirometry. Note the sharp initial peak flow, then relatively straight descent at about 45 degrees to the baseline. There are no stars in the ABN column, indicating that all of the parameters are within normal limits. **B** Mild obstruction. Mild obstruction may be difficult to detect from this spirogram alone. The FEV/FVC% flags this as an obstruction. The severity of the obstruction is mild as judged by the FEV1, which is 78% of the predicted. Mild obstruction occurs gradually over many years.

3. A positive response to bronchodilators is defined as an increase in FVC of 15% or more and an increase in FEV1 of 12% or more.

Postprocedure patient education

Observe patients for fatigue. Inform them the test is over and they may relax.

Practitioner Followup/Complications

Sources of spirometry error and practitioner pitfalls are:

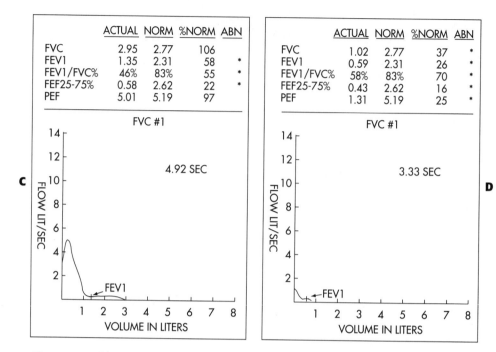

	ACTUAL	NORM	%NORM	ABN
FVC	2.95	2.77	106	
FEV1	1.35	2.31	58	*
FEV1/FVC%	46%	83%	55	*
FEF25-75%	0.58	2.62	22	*
PEF	5.01	5.19	97	

C

FVC #1

4.92 SEC

FEV1

FLOW LIT/SEC — VOLUME IN LITERS

	ACTUAL	NORM	%NORM	ABN
FVC	1.02	2.77	37	*
FEV1	0.59	2.31	26	*
FEV1/FVC%	58%	83%	70	*
FEF25-75%	0.43	2.62	16	*
PEF	1.31	5.19	25	*

D

FVC #1

3.33 SEC

FEV1

FLOW LIT/SEC — VOLUME IN LITERS

Fig. 4-1, cont'd. C Moderate obstruction. The FEV1/FVC is abnormal, indicating obstruc-tion. The FEV1 is 58% of normal, indicating that the obstruction is moderate in severity. Note the concave shape of the flow-volume curve, with low flows after the initially sharp peak flow. **D** Severe obstruction. Severe obstruction with a low vital capacity. All of the parameters are abnormally low. The low FEV1/FVC% indicates obstruction and the FEV1 of only 26% of normal shows that the obstruction is severe. A superimposed restriction may also be present since the FVC is abnormally low, but the patient only tried to exhale for about 3 seconds, so the FVC is probably underestimated. This patient had emphysema.

- Air leak at mouth, nose or device
- Tense patient—cannot take a full breath
- Incomplete emptying of lungs
- Hesitation at the beginning of expiration
- Failure to correct for temperature or humidity
- Recent exposure to inhalants or drugs
- Machine malfunctioning
- Failure to calibrate machine
- Failure to correlate with clinical picture

CPT BILLING CODES
94010—Spirometry, including graphic record, total and timed

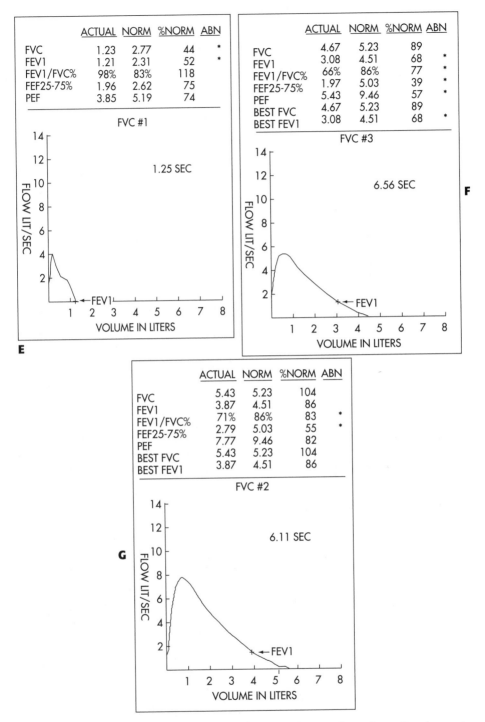

	ACTUAL	NORM	%NORM	ABN
FVC	1.23	2.77	44	*
FEV1	1.21	2.31	52	*
FEV1/FVC%	98%	83%	118	
FEF25-75%	1.96	2.62	75	
PEF	3.85	5.19	74	

FVC #1

1.25 SEC

	ACTUAL	NORM	%NORM	ABN
FVC	4.67	5.23	89	
FEV1	3.08	4.51	68	*
FEV1/FVC%	66%	86%	77	*
FEF25-75%	1.97	5.03	39	*
PEF	5.43	9.46	57	*
BEST FVC	4.67	5.23	89	
BEST FEV1	3.08	4.51	68	*

FVC #3

6.56 SEC

F

	ACTUAL	NORM	%NORM	ABN
FVC	5.43	5.23	104	
FEV1	3.87	4.51	86	
FEV1/FVC%	71%	86%	83	*
FEF25-75%	2.79	5.03	55	*
PEF	7.77	9.46	82	
BEST FVC	5.43	5.23	104	
BEST FEV1	3.87	4.51	86	

FVC #2

6.11 SEC

G

Fig. 4-1, cont'd. **E** Severe restriction. The FEV1/FVC% is normal, so obstruction does not exist. The FVC, however, is only 44% of normal, indicating severe restriction. The FEV1 is also decreased, but to a lesser degree than the FVC in restrictive disorders. Note the sharp peak and rapid, straight, and steep decline of the flow-volume curve. **F** Before bronchodilators. **G** After bronchodilators.

vital capacity, expiratory flow rate measurements.

94060—Bronchospasm evaluation; spirometry before and after bronchodilator.

94160—Vital capacity screening test: total capacity with timed FEV (duration and peak flow rate must be stated).

94375—Respiratory flow-volume loop.

94664—Aerosol or vapor inhalation for sputum mobilization, bronchodilation, or sputum induction for diagnostic purposes; initial demonstration and/or evaluation.

BIBLIOGRAPHY

Altose M, Enright P, Kanner R: Physician's guide to spirometers, *Patient Care* 21:125, 1987.
Crocco J, Kotch A, Neff T: Spirometry: who? when? how? *Patient Care* 25:59, 1991.
Enright P, Hyatt R: *Office spirometry: a practical guide to the selection and use of spirometers,* Philadelphia, 1987, Lea & Febiger.
Enright PL, Lebowitz MD, Cockroft DW: Physiologic measures: pulmonary function tests. Asthma outcome, *Am J Respir Crit Care Med* 149(2, Pt 2):S9, 1994.
Gardner R: Standardization of spirometry: a summary of recommendations from the American Thoracic Society, *Ann Intern Med* 108:217, 1988.
Gillette R: Spirometry. In Gillette R, editor, *Procedures in ambulatory care,* New York, 1987, McGraw-Hill.
Hankinson JL: State of the art of spirometric instrumentation, *Chest* 9(2):258, 1990.
Staff: Does spirometry belong in your office? *Emerg Med* 2:213, 1988.

Oral Airway Insertion

Description

The oropharyngeal airway provides short-term maintenance of a patent airway and prevents the tongue from blocking the upper airway. The oropharyngeal airway is a semicircular device. In the proper position the device will hold the tongue away from the posterior wall of the pharynx. The most frequently used types are plastic and disposable.

Indications

Indications for the insertion of an oral airway are:

- Inspiratory stridor
- Cyanosis
- Unconsciousness
- Seizures

Any time patients are unable to maintain their own patent airway, the oral airway may be indicated, along with proper positioning, until more advanced airway methods can be instituted such as endotracheal intubation. The oral airway can be used short term to maintain a patent airway in patients with signs of upper airway obstruction by the tongue. If the patients are producing snoring sounds (stridor) this could indicate upper airway obstruction. The oral airway can also act as a bite block to prevent damage to the tongue and soft tissue.

Contraindications/Precautions

Practitioners use oral airways only if the patient is unconscious. The insertion of an oral airway in a conscious or semiconscious patient may stimulate vomiting or laryngospasm.

Practitioners may consider the use of a nasopharyngeal airway with the semiconscious patient. A nasopharyngeal airway should not be used if there is trauma to the nose or a suspicion of a basilar skull fracture (blood or CSF from nose or ear).

The proper size airway must be used. If the airway is too large, it will press against the epiglottis, causing total obstruction.

Practitioners should maintain the patient in a side lying position, or with the neck hyperextended (Fig. 4-2, p. 148).

Patient Preparation/Education

The patient should be placed supine, and the head tilt–chin lift used to maintain a patent airway.

Although patients are unconscious, they may be able to hear; the practitioner should tell patients each step of the procedure as it is performed. Patients should be reassured that this will make breathing easier.

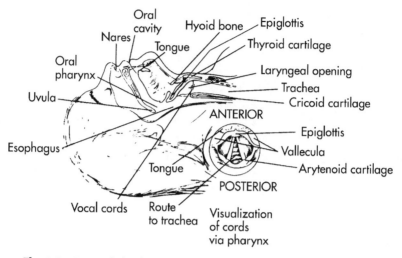

Fig. 4-2 Anatomic landmarks of the head and neck. (From Pfenninger JL, Fowler GC: *Procedures for primary care physicians,* St Louis, 1994, Mosby.)

Equipment

- Oral airway; these range in size to fit infants, children, and adults
- OR nasopharyngeal airway, soft rubber (one size), and water-soluble jelly
- Tongue depressor (optional)
- Suction equipment
- Supplemental oxygen equipment

Procedure

Oropharyngeal airway

1. Place the patient in the supine head tilt position.
2. Choose the correct size of airway by holding airway beside the patient's face; the correct size will extend from the mouth to the angle of the jaw.
3. Hold the airway so that the convex part of the curve faces the top of the patient's head and the tip points toward the roof of the patient's mouth, to avoid pushing the tongue backward.
4. Open the patient's mouth with a tongue blade and advance the tip of the airway along the roof of the mouth (Fig. 4-3).

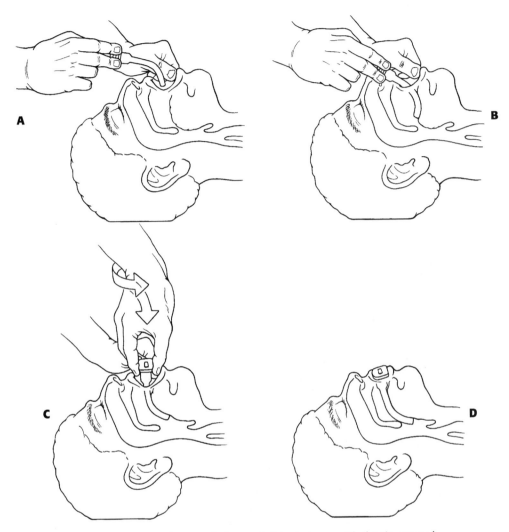

Fig. 4-3 Insertion of an oropharyngeal airway. **A** Orient airway with the tip upward. **B** Advance the tip. **C** Rotate the airway 180 degrees. **D** Airway placed correctly in the oropharynx.

5. Rotate airway 180 degrees so that tip rests in the posterior pharynx.
6. If the patient gags, remove airway immediately and consider using a nasopharyngeal airway.
7. To check for correct placement, auscultate for breath sounds.

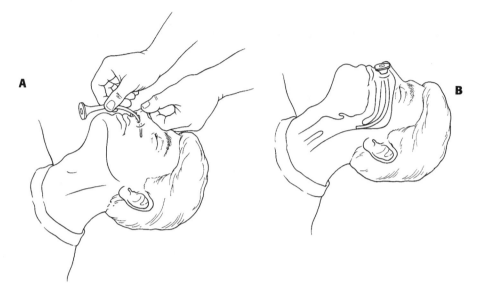

Fig. 4-4 Insertion of a nasopharyngeal airway. **A** Hold airway so its curvature follows the floor of the nose. **B** Slide the airway into the nostril until its flange is flush against the opening of the nostril. Its distal end will then be in the oropharynx.

Nasopharyngeal airway

1. Lubricate the airway with water-soluble jelly.
2. Hold the airway with its tip pointed downward and slide it gently into one nostril (Fig. 4-4).
3. Do not force; if you meet resistance, try the other nostril.

Postprocedure patient education

The patient may experience a sore throat following the procedure. Explain the source of the problem.

Practitioner Followup/Complications

The practitioner should call for help and refer the patient as appropriate.

The practitioner monitors the airway until help arrives.

A proper size and position of the airway is indicated by clear breath sounds.

To prevent trauma, the practitioner should make sure the patient's lips and tongue are not between the teeth and the airway.

The practitioner continues to maintain the side lying or head tilt position to maintain a patent airway.

BIBLIOGRAPHY

American Heart Association: *Textbook of advanced cardiac life support,* Dallas, 1994, Author.

Persons C: *Critical care procedures and protocols,* Philadelphia, 1987, Lippincott.

Caroline NL: *Emergency care in the streets,* ed 4, Boston, 1991, Little, Brown.

CHAPTER 5

Cardiovascular Procedures

Doppler Ultrasound of Lower Extremities

Description

Doppler ultrasound is a noninvasive device used to detect and measure blood flow in major arteries and veins. A hand-held transducer, probe, or flowmeter directs high-frequency sound waves to the artery or vein being tested. The sound waves strike moving red blood cells and are reflected back to the transducer, which then amplifies the sound waves for direct listening and/or graphic recording of blood flow. The tone emitted by the transducer is proportional to the velocity of blood flow in the vessel.

Indications

Doppler ultrasound is used to aid in the diagnosis of chronic venous insufficiency and deep venous thrombosis.

Doppler ultrasound is used to aid in the diagnosis of peripheral arterial insufficiency and arterial occlusion.

It is also used to monitor clients who have had an invasive arterial procedure and or those clients who have undergone arterial reconstruction and bypass grafts.

153

Contraindications/Precautions

Practitioners do not place a doppler probe over an open or draining lesion.

Doppler ultrasound may fail to detect mild arteriosclerotic plaques and smaller thrombi.

Doppler ultrasound may fail to detect major calf vein thrombosis, so the practitioner should be alert for other signs and symptoms.

Doppler ultrasound may fail to detect abnormalities in patients with obese legs or extensive leg swelling.

A cold room will cause vasoconstriction.

Patient Preparation/Education

The practitioner informs the patient that she or he may experience light pressure from the blood pressure cuff and transducer but will not feel the sound waves.

Equipment

- Doppler probe
- Water-soluble conductive jelly
- Sphygmomanometer with arm and thigh cuffs

Procedure

1. Place the patient supine with the head slightly elevated. The patient should be relaxed and comfortable. The patient's legs should be slightly abducted, externally rotated, with knees slightly flexed.
2. Take patient's blood pressure in both arms.
3. Set the volume control on the lowest setting.
4. Apply the conductive gel to the patient's skin.
5. Hold the probe against the skin at a 45 degree angle, pointing toward the heart, over the blood vessel being examined. Use minimal pressure to avoid compressing the blood vessel.
6. Move the probe over the site if flow is not detected, keeping it in direct contact with the skin, and adjust the volume to detect blood flow.

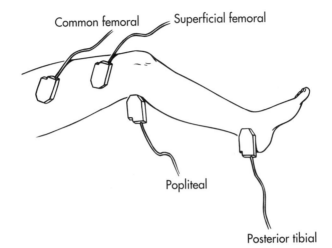

Fig. 5-1 Doppler sonographic examination. The patient is supine with the head slightly elevated. Examine the common femoral, superficial femoral, popliteal, and posterior tibial veins sequentially. (From Pfenninger JL, Fowler GC: *Procedures for primary care physicians,* St Louis, 1994, Mosby.)

7. Evaluate venous flow. Normal venous flow produces a tone that is low pitched and continuous and heard best with the probe pointed toward the heart. Figure 5-1 shows the location of veins accessible to evaluation. Compare the sound from one leg to the other at each site and record.
8. Evaluate arterial flow. Arterial flow produces a high-pitched intermittent tone. Use segmental pressure measurement.
9. Locate and mark the sites where the pulse is heard.
10. Apply the blood pressure cuff at the sites noted in Figure 5-2.
11. Hold the doppler probe over the place where pulse was heard best.
12. Inflate the cuff until the doppler signal in the foot disappears.
13. Deflate the cuff slowly until the first signal is audible, note the pressure, and record this number. Repeat for each site on each leg.

Interpretation of results

Venous flow—normal flow is continuous and equal bilaterally.
Arterial flow—Normal ankle pressure is equal to or slightly greater than the arm pressure. Calculate the ankle-arm pressure index (API) for both ankles by dividing the ankle systolic pres-

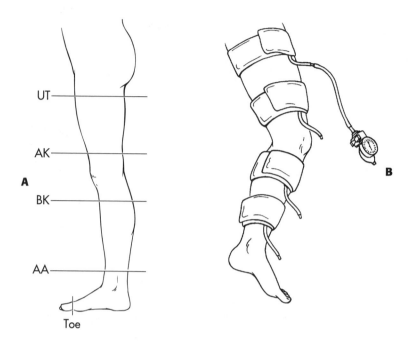

Fig. 5-2 Segmental arterial pressure measurement **A** Cuff positions: UT, upper thigh; AK, above knee; BK, below knee; AA, above ankle. **B** Placement of cuffs. (From Pfenninger JL, Fowler GC: *Procedures for primary care physicians,* St Louis, 1994, Mosby.)

sure by the brachial systolic pressure. An API less than 1.0 is abnormal. Patients with intermittent claudication usually have APIs or 0.5 to 0.9. Patients with rest pain have APIS of less than 0.5.

Postprocedure patient education

For patients with documented venous insufficiency:

Recommend support stockings.

Instruct them to keep their legs elevated whenever possible.

Warn them to avoid constrictive clothing.

Advise female patients to avoid stockings with tight garters.

For patients with documented arterial insufficiency:

Encourage gentle exercise, such as walking, to aid in the development of collateral circulation.

Insist that patients who smoke stop smoking.

If the patient has diabetes mellitus, encourage glycemic control because this may retard the development of peripheral neuropathy.

Encourage dietary control of cholesterol and weight reduction.

In patients with hypertension, insist on control of hypertension to reduce overall cardiovascular mortality.

Practitioner Followup/Complications

The practitioner should consider referral to a vascular surgeon if:

- Ankle pressure is 30 mm Hg or more less than arm systolic pressure.
- The doppler detects an absent pulse (no sound is transmitted).
- There is a neurological deficit in the area being assessed.
- The patient complains of intermittent claudication.
- There are signs and symptoms of infection in the area being assessed, particularly ulcers or blackened tissue.
- There is acute onset of limb-threatening ischemia, which warrants immediate attention of a vascular surgeon. These patients usually presents with severe, acute pain; an absence of pulse; coldness; pallor; and impaired motor and sensory function of the affected limb.

CPT BILLING CODE

93922—Noninvasive physiologic studies of upper or lower extremity arteries, single level, bilateral.

93965—Noninvasive physiologic studies of extremity veins, complete bilateral study.

93970—Duplex scan of extremity veins, including responses to compression and other maneuvers; complete bilateral study.

93971—Followup or limited study.

BIBLIOGRAPHY

Arena L: Flow-augmentation device for peripheral vascular Doppler, *Radiology* 194(1):281, 1995.

Fronek A: *Noninvasive diagnostics in vascular disease,* New York, 1989, McGraw-Hill.

Pfenninger JL, Fowler GC: *Procedures for primary care physicians,* St Louis, 1994, Mosby.

Electrocardiogram

Description

The electrocardiogram (ECG) is a routine, noninvasive diagnostic procedure used to evaluate the electrical activity of the heart in patients with possible cardiovascular disease. Correct lead placement is necessary for an accurate ECG. (See Fig. 5-3.) There are six limb leads, and six precordial leads. Each lead is assigned a polarity. The

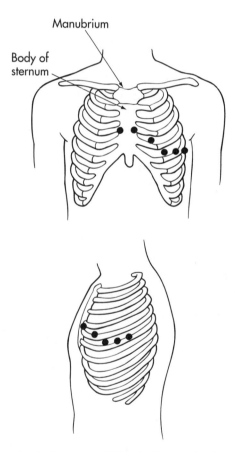

Fig. 5-3 Location of unipolar precordial leads. (From Pfenninger JL, Fowler GC: *Procedures for primary care physicians,* St Louis, 1994, Mosby.)

direction of the current between the polarities will be reflected in the ECG tracing.

Indications

Indications for use of an electrocardiogram are

- Chest pain
- Followup of cardiovascular disease
- Preoperative evaluation
- Differential diagnosis of:
    Ischemic heart disease
    Myocardial infarction
    Cardiomyopathy
    Arrhythmias
    Pericarditis
    Electrolyte abnormalities
    Endocarditis
    Drug toxicity

Contraindications/Precautions

Accurate findings depend on correct lead placement (Fig. 5-3).

It is important that practitioners become familiar with the equipment in their facility. The manufacturer's instruction manual should be read.

A normal ECG does not rule out coronary artery disease.

Patient Preparation/Education

The procedure requires patients to lie still, on their back, for several minutes.

The ECG is noninvasive; it will not hurt or shock.

Equipment

- ECG machine with limb and chest leads and cables
- Proper paper supply

- Electroconductive tags or conduction gel and electrodes
- Grounded safe electrical outlet or charged battery

Procedure

1. Place the patient in a flat supine position.
2. Plug in the machine. Some require a few minutes to warm up.
3. Enter the patient identification according to machine instructions.
4. Set the speed at 25 mm/sec and the sensitivity at 1N.
5. Prepare the skin by cleaning it with an alcohol wipe if it is dirty or oily.
6. Place the conduction gel, then the electrode or electroconductive tags. Figure 5-3 (p. 158) shows the correct placement.

Limb leads

- On the legs, place the electrode on the distal third of the lower legs on the anterior medial surface.
- On the upper extremities place the lead on the volar surfaces of the distal third of the forearms.

Chest leads

- V1—Forth intercostal space at right sternal border
- V2—Fourth intercostal space at left sternal border
- V3—Halfway between V2 and V4
- V4—Fifth intercostal space at the midclavicular line
- V5—Anterior axillary line directly lateral to V4
- V6—Midaxillary line directly lateral to V5

7. Attach the limb and chest lead to the tags as labeled.
8. Record the 12-lead ECG or rhythm strip according to machine instructions.
9. Check the ECG for correct placement of the leads and check for the adequacy of the tracing before removing the leads. If the tracing is distorted, the machine may not be adequately grounded. Recheck and try again.
10. If arrhythmia is noted, obtain a rhythm strip (long lead II).
11. Remove the electrodes and clean the electrogel from the patient and the leads.

Chest Leads Codes

If the machine does not automatically mark the leads, mark them with the code shown below, using the marking button on the ECG machine.

I .
V1 – .
II –
V2 – . .
III – –
V3 – . . .
AVR . . . .
V4 – . . . .
AVL . . . . .
V5 – . . . . .
AVF . . . . . .
V6 – . . . . . .

Interpretation of results

Refer to a text for the basic principles of ECG interpretation. A typical pattern of a normal ECG is included to assist with checking to see if leads have been placed correctly (Fig. 5-4, p. 162).

Postprocedure patient education

Reassure the patient.
Review the results and their implications with the patient.

Practitioner Followup/Complications

You should promptly refer any ECGs suggestive of myocardial infarction, or any abnormalities out of your scope of practice.

Erroneous electrode placement may cause unusual tracings. Check the ECG by looking for erroneous configurations.

CPT BILLING CODES

93000—Electrocardiogram, routine, with at least 12 leads; with interpretation and report.

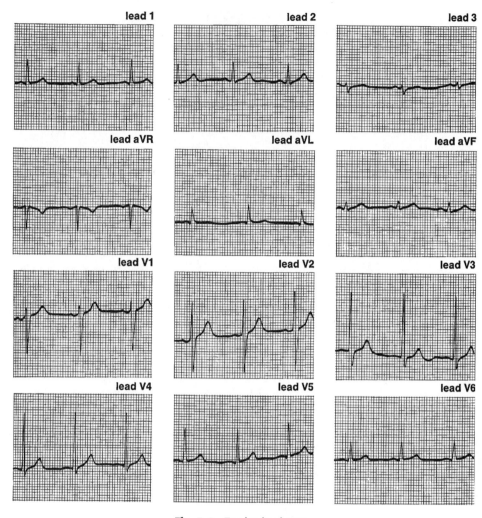

Fig. 5-4 Twelve-lead EKG.

93005—Tracing only, with interpretation and report.
93010—Interpretation and report only.

BIBLIOGRAPHY

Caplan M, Ranieri C: What's his ECG telling you? A guide for nurses, *RN* 52:42, 1989.
Fassler M, Steuble B: *Electrocardiogram interpretation and emergency intervention*, Springhouse, Penn, 1991, Springhouse.
Roberts PW: *Useful procedures in medical practice*, Philadelphia, 1986, Lea & Febiger.

Continuous Electrocardiography (Holter Monitoring)

Description

Holter monitoring involves 24-hour monitoring of a patient's electrocardiogram (ECG). The purpose is to document episodes of abnormal cardiac electrical behavior in the ambulatory patient.

Indications

Use Holter monitoring to evaluate patients with periodic symptoms such as dizziness, palpitations or syncope.

Use Holter monitoring to assess risk in patients with or without symptoms of arrythmia, such as in patients with cardiomyopathies and postinfarction patients with left ventricular dysfunction.

Use Holter monitoring for evaluation of antiarrhythmic drug treatment or pacemaker function.

Use Holter monitoring to assess cardiac status of unreliable subjects who may be unaware of arrhythmia or ectopic beats.

Use Holter monitoring in the diagnosis of obstructive sleep apnea.

Use Holter monitoring to detect myocardial ischemia.

Most monitors utilize a continuous 24-hour recording. Also available are intermittent records, which record only a limited number of episodes, when the patient is experiencing the symptom in question, and a machine that transmits the ECG by telephone. These may be used for patients who experience the target symptom less than once a day.

Contraindications/Precautions

A standard 12-lead ECG should be obtained before ambulatory electrocardiography is done.

Correct placement of the electrodes is necessary, especially for detection of myocardial ischemia.

Caution: This test is expensive, ($200 to $350 in most institutions), so cost should be a consideration when ordering this procedure.

Patient Preparation/Education

Practitioners explain the importance of keeping an event diary.

Practitioners give the patients an event diary with columns for time, symptom or feeling, and activity.

Practitioners instruct the patients to record the time and describe the symptom if they experience the target symptom or any other dizziness, palpitation, syncope, or unusual symptom.

Practitioners instruct the patients to keep a record of the time and their activities even if no symptoms are experienced.

If the patients are unable to keep a diary, the patients should enlist the help of a caregiver.

Practitioners instruct the patients not to take a shower or bath during the 24 hours the monitor is being used.

Equipment

- Holter monitor
- Razor
- Alcohol wipes
- Electrodes, electrode cream
- Lead attachment kit
- Fresh battery

Procedure

Refer to the instruction manual supplied with the machine.

1. Install fresh batteries and a new tape in the machine.
2. Prepare the skin with alcohol wipes.
3. Shave men's skin where electrodes will be placed.
4. Apply electrode cream and then electrodes to the chest as pictured (Fig. 5-5).

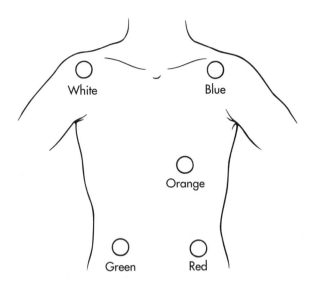

Fig. 5-5   Diagram of lead placement for a Holter monitor.

5. Hook up the leads to the chest.
6. Ensure that the monitor is working correctly by printing out a sample rhythm strip.
7. Put the monitor in its pouch and put the pouch on the patient.
8. Give the patient a diary to take home to record symptoms.
9. Have the patient return in 24 hours to remove the Holter monitor.

Interpretation of results

Interpretation of the results of Holter monitoring is beyond the scope of this book; it requires specialist review and interpretation.

It is important to look for correlations between symptoms and arrhythmias.

Premature ventricular contractions (PVCs) are common in the general population and increase in frequency with increasing age. The presence of PVCs by themselves does not necessarily indicate heart disease.

Postprocedure patient education

Explain the results to the patient.

Practitioner Followup/Complications

Patients should be referred to a physician if significant abnormalities are found on Holter monitoring.

CPT BILLING CODES

93224—Continuous original ECG waveform recording and storage, with visual superimposition scanning; includes recording, scanning, analysis with report, and physician review and interpretation.

93230—Continuous original ECG waveform recording and storage, without superimposition scanning utilizing a device capable of producing a full miniaturized printout; includes recording, microprocessor-based analysis with report, and physician review and interpretation.

93235—Continuous computerized monitoring and noncontinuous recording, and relay-time data analysis utilizing a device capable of producing intermittent full-size waveform tracings, possibly patient activated; includes monitoring and real-time data analysis with report and physician review and interpretation.

BIBLIOGRAPHY

American College of Cardiology/American Heart Association Task Force on Assessment of Diagnostic and Therapeutic Cardiovascular Procedures: Guidelines for ambulatory electrocardiography, *Circulation* 79(1):206, 1989.

Grauer K, Leytem B: A systematic approach to Holter monitor interpretation, *Am Fam Physician* 45:1641, 1992.

Page RL, and others: Asymptomatic arrhythmias in patients with symptomatic paroxysmal atrial fibrillation and paroxysmal supraventricular tachycardia, *Circulation* 89(1):224, 1994.

Pepine CJ: Ambulatory ECG monitoring. How useful in detecting and quantitating transient ischemia? *Postgrad Med* 79(1):141, 1986.

Raby KE, and others: Usefulness of Holter monitoring for detecting myocardial ischemia in patients with nondiagnostic exercise treadmill test, *Am J Cardiol* 72(12):889, 1993.

CHAPTER 6

Gastrointestinal Procedures

Nasogastric Tube Insertion and Removal

Description

Placement of a nasogastric tube (NGT) is a clean procedure used for both diagnosis and therapy. The basic procedures for placing NGT and its removal are described here. Gastric lavage utilizing an NGT is discussed in the following procedure.

Indications

An NGT is used for aspiration of stomach contents.
An NGT is used to administer feedings or medications.

Contraindications/Precautions

Use of an NGT should not be attempted in cases of poisoning with corrosive agents, such as acid and alkali poisoning.
The NGT should not be used for cases of poisoning with hydrocarbons and petroleum distillates.
The procedure should not be attempted if the patient has an acute seizure.

Use of an NGT should not be attempted in a patient with maxillofacial or skull trauma.

Esophageal perforations and submucosal passage of the NGT are more likely to occur if the NGT is forced during advancement. Aspiration potential can be decreased by maintaining the head of the bed at greater than 30 degrees. Mucosal ulcerations of the nose, pharynx, and stomach are less likely to occur if the tube is periodically rotated and irrigated and the tube is secured in place without placing pressure on the nose. Pressure occurs when the tube is sharply bent upwards as soon as it exits the nostril and is taped down over the nose. Proper placement of the NGT should be ascertained before any solutions are administered. Head flexion and slow advancement timed with the patient's repeated swallowing helps prevent the NGT from entering the larynx and lungs. Using a water-soluble lubricant decreases the risk for lung infection should it be aspirated. Keep the patient NPO and place the patient in a semi- to high Fowler's position for aspiration and lavage.

Patient Preparation/Education

Sensations likely to be experienced include gagging (with possible vomiting), tearing, and nasal discomfort. Practitioners should review the methods used to ease NG tube insertion with patient, for example, mouth breathing, swallowing, head hyperextension, and flexion. Practitioners reassure the patient that tissues and an emesis basin are readily available for use as needed.

Equipment

- Nasogastric tube (No. 6, 8, or 12 Levin or No. 14 to 16 French for an adult, a No. 10 French for a child)
- Water-soluble lubricant or 2% viscous lidocaine gel
- Penlight or flashlight
- Waterproof pad or towel
- Stethoscope
- 1-inch hypoallergenic cloth tape
- Safety pin (optional)
- Rubber band (optional)

- Tissues
- Two plastic emesis basins (one for ice or water in which to soak the NGT, and one in which to empty gastric contents)
- A 60-ml catheter tip syringe with piston
- Clean gloves
- Goggles (optional)
- Glass of water and straw (optional)
- Connecting tubing and suction equipment (optional)
- pH paper (optional)
- Clamp for NGT (optional)
- One or two 1-L bottles of sterile normal saline irrigating solution

Procedure

1. If the NGT is rubber, place it in the plastic basin on ice for at least 5 minutes before insertion. This will increase the tube's rigidity, allowing easier advancement. If the NGT is plastic, however, place it in the basin in warm water. This increases the tube's pliability, making its insertion easier.
2. Place a waterproof pad or towel across the patient's chest and, if possible, elevate the head of the bed at least 45 degrees.
3. Remove any ill-fitting dentures.
4. Have the patient hyperextend his or her head. Use the penlight or flashlight to observe the nostrils for patency. In addition, occlude each nostril separately and have the patient breathe through the unoccluded nostril. Select the nostril with better airflow for NGT insertion.
5. Estimate the distance the NGT will need to be inserted for it to reach the stomach by placing the distal end of the NGT at the tip of the nose, extending the tube across to the tip of the earlobe, and then continuing on to the tip of the sternum's xiphoid process. Mark the site on the tube using tape.
6. Lubricate the first 4 inches of the NGT with the water-soluble jelly and coil the tube around your fingers for a few seconds to help stiffen the tube for easier insertion. In addition, using a topical anesthetic in the nostril or oropharynx can aid in insertion.

7. With the patient's head upright to hyperextended, insert the distal end of the tube into the nostril with the tube curvature following the natural curvature at the nasopharyngeal junction. Gently advance the NGT along the nostril floor and downward toward the patient's ipsilateral ear until the oropharynx is reached. This is when resistance and gagging are encountered (Fig. 6-1).

8. At this point, have the patient flex his or her head slightly forward and rotate the tube inward 180 degrees toward the contralateral nostril. Have the patient begin swallowing repeatedly (if the patient isn't NPO, give him or her the glass of water and straw from which to drink) as the tube is slowly being advanced. Time advancement attempts with the swallows so that no more than 3 to 5 inches of tubing are advanced with each swallow. Too rapid advancements can lead to NGT coiling in the oropharynx and coming out the mouth. Keep in mind that resistance may be encountered on NGT advancement behind the cricoid cartilage, behind the bifurcation of the bronchus, and at the esophagogastric sphincter.

9. Whenever the patient starts to gag, stop advancing briefly and observe for NGT coiling in the oropharynx or signs of respiratory distress. If any signs of respiratory distress such as dyspnea or inability to talk occur, withdraw the tube and reattempt insertion when the patient is out of respiratory distress. When excessive gagging is encountered, have the patient breathe or take small sips of water without advancing the tube to calm down the gag reflex.

10. Continue advancing the NGT once the gag reflex has diminished as previously described until the tape mark on the tube reaches the tip of the nose. At this point temporarily secure the tube in place with tape and check for correct placement of the NGT.

11. First aspirate a small amount of fluid to determine whether there are gastric contents present. The fluid should be clear to yellow with mucus and have a pH less than 7. Gastric contents may be difficult if not impossible to aspirate when small-bore NGTs are inserted.

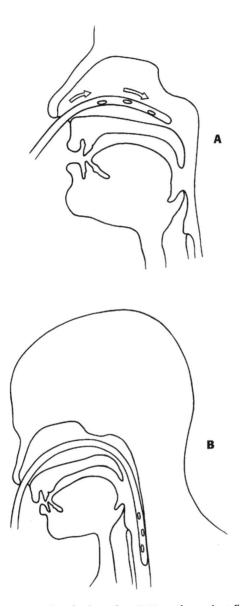

Fig. 6-1 **A** Nasogastric tube insertion. **B** Have the patient flex the head and gently advance the tube, then ask the patient to swallow. (From Pfenninger JL, Fowler GC: *Procedures for primary care physicians,* St Louis, 1994, Mosby.)

12. Next, using the plastic syringe, draw up 10 ml of air, attach the syringe to the proximal end of the NGT, and place the diaphragm of the stethoscope over the epigastric/stomach area. Instill the 10 ml of air and, using the stethoscope, auscultate for a swooshing sound or rush of air indicating that the tube is likely in the stomach.

13. Then, either leave the syringe attached to the proximal end of the NGT and clamp the NGT, or attach it to suction.

14. Tear off a 4-inch piece cloth tape and split 2 inches of it vertically. Replace the temporary tape with this tape by placing the unsplit end over the bridge of the nose and wrapping the chevron ends underneath and around the NGT in opposite directions while keeping the NGT straight downwards from the nose.

15. Complete the NGT securing by wrapping a piece of cloth tape or the rubber band around the tube near the proximal end and pinning it to the patient's gown or clothing.

16. Proceed with any other necessary procedures such as gastric emptying, lavage, medication, or feeding administration.

17. Maintain the NGT by periodically rotating and retaping the tube to minimize the potential for mucosal necrosis; keep the mouth, throat, and nostrils moist by using room humidity, throat lozenges or sprays, gum, or hard candy; and clean the nostrils and mouth and apply lubricant to the nostrils frequently. Note the amount, color, consistency, and presence of heme or clots in the gastric drainage/aspirate, residual volumes, and any resistance encountered on flushing or instilling solutions. Note the presence of any abdominal distention, bowel sounds, bowel movements, flatus, nausea, vomiting, and abdominal pain.

Criteria for removal of an NGT

There is a decrease in nasogastric drainage.

The patient has normoactive bowel sounds or flatus.

The patient shows absence of abdominal distention.

The patient shows ability to tolerate the NGT clamped or to straight drainage without nausea, vomiting, or abdominal distention.

The patient can tolerate sips of clear liquids without nausea, vomiting, or abdominal distention.

The patient can swallow without difficulty.

The patient is mentally awake and alert with gag present.

The practitioner has completed the required procedures, e.g., lavage.

Removal of the nasogastric tube

1. Explain to patient the rationale for removing the NGT, its basic method, and the likely sensations to be experienced during removal of the NGT.
2. Place the patient in a semi-Fowler's position with an absorbent towel or pad over his or her chest, and don clean gloves.
3. Instill a small amount of normal saline solution into the NGT to free it from the lining of the stomach. Then, using the nondominant hand, fold over the proximal end of the NGT and hold it tightly pinched so that it is clamped off.
4. Ask the patient to flex the head forward, take a deep breath, and hold it. Then steadily and quickly withdraw the NGT and dispose of it.
5. Allow the patient to breathe upon removal of the NGT and provide tissues and an emesis basin for the sneezing, tearing, coughing, and gagging that is likely to ensue immediately after removal.
6. Monitor the patient for the next 48 hours for nausea, vomiting, abdominal distention, and food intolerance.

Practitioner Followup/Complications

Practitioners should assess for the development of submucosal, intracranial, or pulmonary passage of the NGT, esophageal perforation, mucosal ulcerations of the nose, pharynx, or stomach, and aspiration of stomach contents into the lungs leading to pneumonia.

CPT BILLING CODE

9110—Intestinal feeding tube, passage, positioning, and monitoring.

91105—Gastric intubation and aspiration or lavage for treatment (ingested poisons).

BIBLIOGRAPHY

Camp D, Otten, N: How to insert and remove nasogastric tubes, *Nursing* 20(9):59, 1990.
Cockrell C, Cho S: Placement of enteric feeding tubes using guidewire technique, *Southern Med J* 78(2):210, 1985.
Dees, G: Difficult nasogastric tube insertions, *Emerg Med Clin North Am* 7(1):177, 1989.
Eisenberg PG: Nasoenteral tubes, *RN* 57(10):62, 1994.
Methany N: Minimizing respiratory complications of nasoenteric tube feedings: state of the science, *Heart & Lung* 22(3):213, 1993.
Varella L: Nasoenteral tube feeding. In Rombeau JL, and others, editors: *Atlas of nutritional support techniques,* Boston, 1989, Little Brown.

Gastric Lavage

Description

Gastric lavage is the washing from the stomach of its contents, i.e., blood and toxins, for purposes of arresting bleeding or decreasing the systemic absorption of poisonous substances. Ipecac syrup (15 ml for children, 30 ml for adults) is often used for known toxic ingestion. Ipecac is contraindicated in patients who are semiconscious, who are unconscious, or who may have seizures (to avoid aspiration). In these patients, lavage is indicated. Medications

---

Medications Bound by Activated Charcoal

Aspirin
Dextroamphetamine
Strychnine
Chloroquine
Phenytoin
Phenobarbital
Theorphylline
Tricyclic antidepressants
Primaquine phosphate
Glutethimide

bound by activated charcoal are listed in the box.

Lavage is also used to prepare the stomach for a diagnostic procedure or to obtain gastric washing specimens for analysis.

Indications

Indications for gastric lavage are:

- Upper gastrointestinal (GI) bleeding
- Poisoning with a noncorrosive agent
- Drug overdose
- Acquisition of fresh gastric washing specimens for cystology and analysis
- Preparation for diagnostic testing, e.g., endoscopy

Contraindications/Precautions

Gastric lavage should not be attempted in cases of poisoning with corrosive agents, e.g., acid and alkali poisoning and poisoning with hydrocarbons and petroleum distillates. This contraindication also applies for Ipecac.

The procedure should not be attempted if the patient has an acute seizure.

Proper placement of the NGT should be ascertained before administration of any solutions.

Patient Preparation/Education

Practitioners perform baseline laboratory work to include a CBC, electrolytes, type and cross (in suspected upper GI bleeding), and toxicology screens (in suspected drug overdose or poisoning). Practitioners complete a medical history and a physical examination to determine potential sites of bleeding and ascertain the type of poison ingested. Relevant past and present medical history should be ascertained, e.g., congestive heart failure (CHF). The patient should be kept NPO and placed in a semi- to high Fowler's position for aspiration and lavage.

Sensations likely to be experienced include gagging (with possible vomiting) and nasal discomfort.

Equipment

- Nasogastric tube (No. 6, 8, or 12 Levin or a No. 14 to 16 French for an adult, No. 10 French for child)
- Equipment to insert tube—see Procedure on NGT insertion.
- Two plastic emesis basins (one for ice or water in which to cool the normal saline for GI bleed, and one in which to empty gastric contents). Do not use ice with children because it can cause hypothermia.
- A 60-ml catheter tip syringe with piston
- Clean gloves
- Connecting tubing and suction equipment (optional)
- pH paper (optional)
- Clamp for the NGT (optional)
- One or two 1-L bottles of sterile normal saline irrigating solution
- Any antidotes, absorbents, or cathartics indicated
- Activated charcoal (1 gm/kg) for poisonings

Procedure

1. Place NGT—see Procedure on NGT placement.
2. Check for correct placement of the NGT: First aspirate a small amount of fluid to determine whether it is gastric contents and obtain a specimen. The fluid should be clear to yellow with mucus and a pH less than 7. Gastric contents may be difficult if not impossible to aspirate when small-bore NGTs are placed. Aspiration is done by pulling back on the syringe piston after connecting it to the proximal portion of the NGT.

   Using the plastic syringe, draw up 10 ml of air, attach the syringe to the proximal end of the NGT, and place the diaphragm of the stethoscope over the epigastric/stomach area. Instill the 10 ml of air and, using the stethoscope, auscultate for a swooshing sound or rush of air indicating the tube is likely to be in the stomach. Then either leave the syringe attached to the proximal end of the NGT and clamp the NGT, or attach it to suction.
3. Secure the NG tube: Tear off a 4-inch piece of cloth tape and split 2 inches of it vertically. Replace the temporary tape with this tape by placing the unsplit end over the bridge of the nose

and wrapping the chevron ends underneath and around the
NGT in opposite directions while keeping the NGT straight
downwards from the nose.

Finish securing the NGT by wrapping a piece of cloth tape or
the rubber band around the tube near the proximal end and
pinning it to the patient's gown or clothing.

4. Proceed with the lavage:
   a. Instill the iced saline in 50 to 60 ml increments up to a maximum of 200 ml before aspirating back or suctioning out the stomach contents. Overfilling of the stomach can lead to regurgitation and/or aspiration of the instilled solution and stomach contents.
   b. Be sure to let the cool solution sit in the stomach for a least a minute or two before aspirating or suctioning so that the vasoconstriction desired to arrest the bleeding may occur.
   c. Continue the process until the returns are essentially clear.
5. When the lavage is complete, the stomach may be left empty or an antidote, cathartic, or absorbent may be instilled as indicated by the underlying causative poisonous agent. Cathartics facilitate the poison's transition through the intestines, whereas absorbents are instilled to limit the amount of absorption of the poison.

Practitioner Followup/Complications

During and after the lavage, the practitioners monitor the patient's vital signs, hydration, mental, renal, respiratory, and cardiovascular status and administer IV fluids and blood products as necessary.

In cases of poisoning, practitioners should pay particular attention to signs and symptoms of mucosal destruction, i.e., increased burning and pain, drooling, and dysphagia.

Practitioners monitor the patient for the next 48 hours for nausea, vomiting, abdominal distention, and food intolerance.

CPT BILLING CODE

91100—Intestinal bleeding tube, passage, positioning, and monitoring.

91105—Gastric intubation, and aspiration or lavage for treatment (e.g., for ingested poisons).

BIBLIOGRAPHY

Basuk PM, Isenberg JI: Gastric lavage in patients with gastrointestinal hemorrhage. Yea or nay? *Arch Intern Med* 150(7):1379, 1990.
Mertes JE: Action Stat! B.I. Bleeding, *Nursing* 19(8):37, 1989.
Rodgers GC Jr, Matyunas NJ: Gastrointestinal decontamination for acute poisoning, *Pediatr Clin North Am* 33(2):261, 1986.
Wojner AW: Seconds count when a child is poisoned, *RN* 56(10):46, 1993.

Anoscopy

Description

Anoscopy can be used to evaluate the patient with perianal and anal complaints.

Indications

Indications for anoscopy

- Anal or perianal pain
- Rectal prolapse (see Procedure on reduction)
- Hemorrhoids

Contraindications/Precautions

Practitioners need to proceed with caution in a patient with an acute cardiovascular condition.

Anoscopy would not be attempted in a patient with an acute abdomen.

Patient Preparation/Education

Practitioners should explain that this procedure will be uncomfortable, but should not be very painful, and give the patient an estimate of the total time for the procedure.

Equipment

- Anoscope
- Light source
- Gloves
- Lubricant
- Cotton swabs

Procedure

1. Position the patient in the left lateral decubitus position and drape (Fig. 6-2, A).
2. Examine the perianal area.
3. Have the patient bear down. Observe for prolapse of hemorrhoids, or rectum.
4. Perform a digital rectal exam.
5. Lubricate the anoscope with the obturator in place.
6. Insert the anoscope slowly in the direction of the umbilicus.
7. Remove the obturator.
8. Observe the mucosa; remove fecal material with a swab.
9. Remove the anoscope slowly, observing the mucosa.

Postprocedure patient education

Discuss findings and followup plans with the patient.

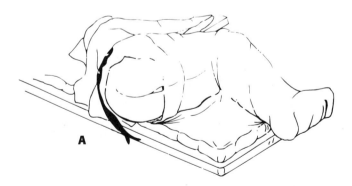

A

Fig. 6-2 A Placing the patient in the left lateral decubitus position (Sim's position). Digital examination, flexible sigmoidoscopy, and most anorectal procedures can be performed in this position.

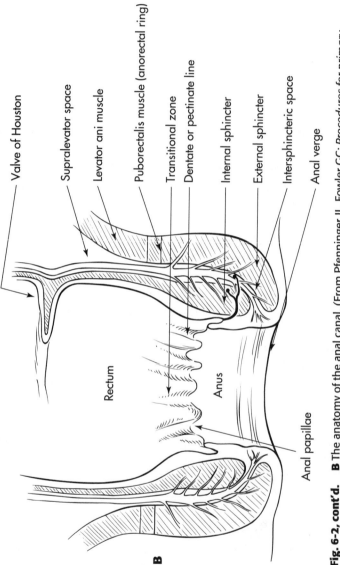
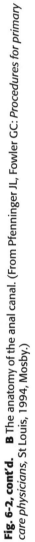

Valve of Houston

Supralevator space

Levator ani muscle

Puborectalis muscle (anorectal ring)

Transitional zone

Dentate or pectinate line

Internal sphincter

External sphincter

Intersphincteric space

Anal verge

Rectum

Anus

Anal papillae

B

Fig. 6-2, cont'd. **B** The anatomy of the anal canal. (From Pfenninger JL, Fowler GC: *Procedures for primary care physicians*, St Louis, 1994, Mosby.)

Practitioner Followup/Complications

Patients should be evaluated for abrasion or tearing of perianal skin or mucosa, or hemorrhoidal tissue. Some small amount of bleeding may occur.

CPT BILLING CODES
46600—Anoscopy.

BIBLIOGRAPHY
Farmer KC, Church JM: Open sesame: tips for traversing the anal canal, *Dis Colon Rectum* 35(11):1092, 1992.
Pfenninger JL, Fowler GC: *Procedures for primary care physicians*, St Louis, 1994, Mosby.

Rectal Prolapse Reduction

Description

Prolapse is a protrusion of the rectum through the anus. The types of rectal prolapse are listed in the box.

Complete rectal prolapse is a relatively rare but serious disorder most often seen in infants or elderly individuals. It is more

---

Types of Rectal Prolapse

Partial: The rectal mucosa protrudes for 1-3 cm beyond the anal sphincter. In mucosal prolapse, the mucosal folds are radial, the anus is inverted and there is no sulcus groove between the anus and the protruding tissue.

Complete: There is an intussusception of all three layers of the rectum through the anal opening. The mucosal folds are concentric, the anus is in a normal anatomical position, and there is a sulcus between the anus and the protruding bowel tissue.

Internal: Patients have symptoms of rectal prolapse but tissue cannot be demonstrated to protrude through the anal canal.

common in women than in men. Factors that predispose rectal prolapse include:

- Chronic constipation
- Severe chronic diarrhea
- Obstetrical injury
- Neurological disease, such as multiple sclerosis
- Weakness of the external rectal sphincter
- Rectal intercourse, including sexual abuse

Indications

Practitioners should rule out conditions that may be confused with rectal prolapse: hemorrhoids, mucosal prolapse, polyps in the lower rectum, and cancer.

Diagnosis is made on inspection and demonstrating the prolapse.

The presence of pain indicates incarceration with impending strangulation or some other condition not related to the prolapse.

Patients with complete rectal prolapse should be referred after reduction for proctoscopy and barium enema or endoscopy to confirm the diagnosis and exclude other lesions. Children should be carefully evaluated to rule out sexual abuse. Once a complete rectal prolapse is diagnosed, conservative methods should be initially tried before surgical intervention. When episodes of recurrences increase and the tissue become prone to excoriation and ulcerations and at risk for strangulation, surgery should be considered. However, the surgical options so far are not extremely successful in preventing or alleviating fecal incontinence.

If the prolapse is small and limited to the mucosa, a high-residue diet and reeducation on bowel habits to prevent straining may control the problem.

Equipment

- Sterile gauze
- Normal saline
- Chux pads/tissues
- Anoscope
- Water-soluble lubricant

Procedure

1. Place patients in a left lateral position. Have tissues available for patients if they report urinary stress incontinence.
2. Ask patients to strain. This pressure should reveal a full thickness rectal prolapse as it mushrooms through the anal sphincters.
3. If straining does not produce a prolapse, have patients squat or have them sit on the toilet to produce the prolapse.
4. Differentiate between hemorrhoid, mucosal (partial) prolapse, or rectal (complete) prolapse by visual exam.
5. Assist patients into a left lateral decubitus position—side lying on left, knee to chest position: This position allows the abdominal viscera to fall cephalad, which may pull the extruded bowel back through the anus and reduce the prolapse.
6. Place a saline-soaked gauze over the prolapse to prevent it from drying.
7. Apply very gentle pressure with the saline-moistened gauze to guide the protruding tissue through the relaxed sphincter.
8. Perform a rectal exam to note sphincter tone at rest and with voluntary contraction. The exam should be painless. Pain should raise suspicion of incarceration or an unrelated lesion.
9. Apply lubricant to the anoscope and insert slowly anteriorly. Remove the inner cannula. Slowly withdraw the anoscope. Identify lesions. It is rare to see a polyp or carcinoma. More likely seen are erythema and edema at the distal 8 to 10 cm, particularly anteriorly.

Postprocedure patient education

Teach the patient or the caregiver the above positioning and pressure application procedure of reduction in the event that the prolapse recurs.

Advise the patient that efforts should be focused on preventing recurrent prolapse, which will lead to continuous prolapse, fecal incontinence, and surgery.

Instruct the patient to increase fiber in the diet. Fiber absorbs water and increases stool bulk, stimulating peristalsis and bowel emptying. Uncooked fruits and vegetables are good sources of bulk. Cereal fiber is a more effective stool softener than fruits and vegetables. Prunes have a laxative effect in some people.

Also instruct the patient that 2000 to 2500 cc per day of fluid intake will help keep the stool soft. Space the fluid at intervals throughout the day so that it does not diminish the appetite.

Advise the patient to select a consistent time of day to attempt defecation. The gastrocolic reflex that occurs 20 to 40 minutes after eating would make this an optimal time. Also, the gastro-colic reflex is stronger after a hot meal, so that a regular habit may be established after a hot breakfast or dinner rather than following a regular cold lunch. Since the optimal physiological position for defecation is the squat, those patients who must use a built-up toilet seat should be advised to elevate their feet on a foot rest and bend forward when attempting a bowel movement.

If these measures do not relieve constipation, order a bulk-forming laxative such as Metamucil or a stool softener such as Colace to facilitate stool transit through the colon.

Practitioner Followup/Complications

The practitioner should make a followup referral for rectal pro-lapse considered to be either partial or complete. Patients may be instructed that they may anticipate biopsy, sigmoidoscopy, or a barium enema for a complete evaluation.

If conservative therapy is recommended to patients with a complete prolapse, anal sphincter function should be assessed regularly to ensure there is no deterioration.

Practitioners assess for complications by noting progression: increases in recurrences, decreasing anal sphincter tone, the development of fecal incontinence, or the presence of pain.

Practitioners should refer for surgical intervention if the patient's condition deteriorates.

After surgical intervention the patient should be observed for the following complications: hemorrhage, bowel obstruction, pelvic abscess, fecal impaction, and recurrent prolapse.

BIBLIOGRAPHY

Buls J: Rectal prolapse. In Fazio VW, editor: *Current therapy in colon and rectal surgery,* Philadelphia, 1990, B.C. Decker.

Gillies D: Nursing care for aged patients with rectal prolapse, *J Gerontol Nurs* 11(2):29, 1985.

Keighley M, and others: Rectal prolapse. In Henry MM, Swash M, editors: *Colo-proctology and the pelvic floor,* Boston, 1992, Butterworth-Heinemann.

Nichols J, Glass R: *Coloproctology: diagnosis and outpatient management,* New York, 1985, Springer-Verlag.

Percutaneous Endoscopic Gastrostomy Tube (PEG) Management

Description

A percutaneous endoscopic gastrostomy tube (PEG) is placed as a same-day surgical procedure (Fig. 6-3). There are an infinite variety of PEGs. Many have a tube that must be clamped. Some have a "button" that can be used to close the tube between uses (Fig. 6-4). The button is a small, flexible silicone device that has a mushroom-type dome at one end and two small wings at the other end. There is a one-way valve inside the device to prevent reflux of stomach contents. The PEG is used for long-term enteral feeding in a patient unable to take adequate oral nutrition. See Nasogastric Tube procedure for information on how to feed a patient using an NGT or a PEG tube. This procedure discusses the care of a PEG tube.

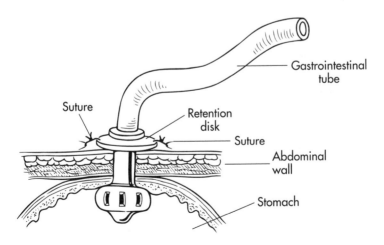

Fig. 6-3 Percutaneous endoscopic gastrostomy tube.

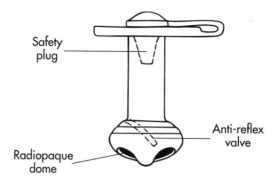

Safety plug

Anti-reflex valve

Radiopaque dome

Fig. 6-4 Gastrostomy feeding button.

Indications

A PEG is used for long-term enteral nutrition.

A PEG is more cosmetically esthetic than conventional gastrostomy or NGTs and is accompanied by fewer complications.

Contraindications/Precautions

PEGs should not be used in the presence of:

- A nonfunctional GI tract
- A paralytic ileus
- A gastric outlet obstruction

There may be an inability to perform the procedure because of

- Gastric or duodenal ulceration
- Severely scarred abdominal wall
- Significant ascites
- Morbid obesity
- Sepsis
- Coagulopathy
- Peritoneal dialysis

Patient Preparation/Education

Practitioners should have the patients lie on their back in bed with their head slightly elevated.

Practitioners show the patients the equipment and explain the procedure, its risks, and its benefits.

Equipment

- Gastrostomy feeding button
- Water based lubricant
- 8 to 10 French catheter
- Normal saline
- Hydrogen peroxide
- Cotton swab

Procedure

The PEG is performed by a surgeon.

Postprocedure patient education

Give nothing via tube for 24 hours postinsertion.

After 24 hours, give plain water, followed with formula if it is tolerated.

Leave the original dressing in place for 48 hours.

After 48 hours, for the next 2 weeks, clean the insertion with half-strength hydrogen peroxide and cotton swab; then wipe it with a cotton swab soaked with sterile normal saline and apply a sterile dressing.

After 2 weeks, use clean technique to clean with soap and water; do not apply a dressing. Rotate the tube in a full circle while cleaning. Allow for complete drying, with the patient's skin exposed to air for 20 minutes. The patient can be fully immersed in water.

Flush the button with 5 to 10 cc of water after feeding or medication administration

Clean the inside tube with a cotton-tip applicator and water to maintain patency and reduce bacterial growth.

Practitioner Followup/Complications

Dislodgment of button

1. The button should be saved for reinsertion. This is not a medical emergency. The stoma will remain open for several hours.

2. The practitioner slightly lubricates the obturator, the dome of the button, and the stoma site with a water-soluble lubricant.
3. The obturator is pushed down the shaft of the button to distend it. Then the distended button is inserted into the stoma.
4. If it is not possible to reinsert the button, refer.

Leakage of stomach contents caused by failure of the antireflux valve of the button

1. The obturator or an 8 to 10 French suction catheter should be gently inserted into the shaft of the button until it moves the valve back to the closed position.
2. The antireflux valve will make a popping sound and the stomach contents will stop leaking.

Redness and irritation around the stoma

This may cause skin complications: maceration, fungal infection, or pressure necrosis.

1. The practitioner should clean the stoma site with half-strength hydrogen peroxide followed with Betadine.
2. Stomahesive powder is then applied.
3. The stoma site should be cleaned more frequently.
4. The stoma site should be well dried and left exposed to air for 20 to 30 minutes.
5. If formula or milk is spilled on the skin, it should be cleaned off immediately.

Plugging of the button or PEG

Occlusion may develop from food and/or medication. To prevent:

1. Liquid medications or well-ground, diluted medication should be used.
2. The button should be irrigated with 5 to 10 cc of tap water after food and medication have been administered. Irrigate the PEG with 25 to 50 cc of tap water after administration of food or medicine.
3. The inside of the feeding button should be cleaned with tap water and a cotton-tipped applicator to help maintain patency.

Removal of plug

1. The practitioner attaches a 10 cc syringe with 2 to 3 cc of air or water and gently tries to dislodge the plug.
2. Practitioner inserts an 8 or 10 French suction catheter about 1 inch into the shaft of the button and gently tries to push the plug through.
3. Alternate methods for unplugging PEGs include irrigation with a cola drink and insertion of a guide wire. Use a guide wire with caution since it can perforate the tube.

Gastritis

The patient complains of indigestion.

1. Smaller more frequent feedings may help.
2. A histamine blocker such as ranitidine (Zantac) syrup (15 mg/ 1 ml) 150 mg should be administered via the tube daily. Dose should be adjusted for children.

Gastroesophageal reflux with aspiration

To prevent:

1. The practitioner elevates the head of the bed 45 to 60 degrees during feeding and 1 hour after feeding. The practitioner watches for the development of sacral pressure sores.
2. Smaller more frequent feedings may help.

Tube migration

This can cause pyloric obstruction or mucosal perforation.

1. The practitioner measures the length of the tube; if the length is decreasing, the tube is migrating inward.
2. The practitioner may consider medication to decrease gastric motility.

Diarrhea

1. The practitioner should look for other causes of diarrhea such as *C. difficile.*
2. The practitioner should slow the tube feeding time.
3. The practitioner can change patient to another feeding, with fiber in it.

BIBLIOGRAPHY

Bockus S: When your patient needs tube feedings: making the right decisions, *Nursing 93* 23(7):34, 1993.

Huth M, O'Brien M: The gastrostomy feeding tube, *Pediatr Nurs* 13(4):24, 1987.

Methany N, and others: How to aspirate fluid from small-bore feeding tubes, *Am J Nurs* 93(5):86, 1993.

Perry AG, Potter PA: *Clinical nursing skills and techniques,* ed 3, St Louis, 1994, Mosby.

Vautier G, Scott BB: Blocked gastrostomy tubes, *Lancet* 343(8905):1105, 1994.

Enteral Tube Feeding

Description

Some patients require enteral tube feedings to obtain necessary nutrients. Malnutrition comprises a ganglioglioma of clinical conditions that arise from abnormalities associated with nutrient intake, digestion, absorption, metabolism, and excretion. The maximum period of 7 days for severely limited intake is the empirical limit most investigators set for hospitalized patients.

Most investigations indicate that significant weight loss is more than 10% of preillness weight. Weight loss exceeding 10% to 20% is usually accompanied by functional abnormalities and poor clinical outcome.

When malnutrition with depletion of body cell mass and impaired tissue and organ function is not treated, weakness, compromised immunity, decreased wound healing, and complications are more likely to occur. Total absence of enteral nutrition leads to atrophy of the mucosal lining of the small intestine within a few days. This can lead to bacterial translocation, sepsis, and multiple organ failure, resulting in high morbidity. This produces suboptimal response to medical and surgical therapies.

Indications

Tube feeding is indicated for those who will not eat or should not eat and have a functional GI tract:

- Anorexia disorders

- Neurological injury or disease
- Psychiatric disorders such as depression
- Cachexia secondary to cancer, cardiac, and pulmonary disease
- Burns and trauma
- Profound mental retardation or cerebral palsy

Tube feedings may also be indicated for mechanical GI tract dysfunction:

- Facial/jaw injuries
- Head and neck cancer
- Dysphagia
- Benign obstruction of the upper gut

Metabolic GI tract dysfunction may also necessitate tube feedings:

- Pancreatitis
- Inflammatory bowel disease
- Blind loop syndrome
- Multiple food allergies

Some hypermetabolic conditions may also be an indication for tube feedings:

- Major burns
- Major trauma
- Sepsis
- Major surgery

Route selection depends on the anticipated duration of feeding, the condition of the GI tract (esophageal obstruction, prior gastric or small bowel resections), and the potential for aspiration.

Nasogastric, nasoduodenal, and nasojejunal feeding route are possible. Nasogastric feeding is the simplest and most often used method and is preferred for those patients who are expected to resume oral feedings. Access to the duodenum and jejunum is possible with longer, weighted tubes for patients at higher risk for aspiration.

Gastrostomy, jejunostomy, or percutaneous endoscopic gastric tube feedings are indicated when long-term feeding is anticipated or when obstruction makes nasal intubation impossible. Jejunostomy allows for earlier postoperative feedings because the small bowel is less affected than the stomach or colon by postoperative ileus.

Contraindications/Precautions

Practitioners do not attempt these procedures in patients with:

- Nonfunctional GI tract
- Intractable vomiting
- Intestinal obstruction
- Upper GI bleeding
- Severe risk of aspiration

Pulmonary aspiration of the feeding formula is the most serious and life-threatening complication. Vomiting and pulmonary aspiration are most likely to occur when gastric emptying is delayed. The risk can be lessened by elevating the upper body to at least 30 degrees, positioning the tube well below the pylorus—ideally into the proximal small intestine, and frequently testing for gastric residual.

Enteral tube feedings are considered safer than parenteral feedings, because mechanical, infectious, and metabolic complications are usually less severe.

When gastric emptying is delayed, pharmacological intervention with metaclopramide may be tried.

Enteral feeding in patients with end-stage dementia who have decreased food intake is usually a futile procedure that causes patients more distress than benefit. Practitioners should always consider the overall prognosis of the patient and the goals of therapy before starting enteral feedings.

Patient Preparation/Education

The procedure should be pain free.
The patient should expect to feel full after feedings.

Equipment

- Feeding tube, 36 inch for stomach, 43 inch for duodenum/ jejunum
- Guide wire (optional)
- 50-ml syringes with appropriate tip
- Stethoscope
- Litmus paper

Procedure

1. Before initiating feeding ascertain the position of the tube. If it is not possible to aspirate gastric contents, confirm the position with an abdominal x-ray examination. X-ray exam confirmation must be done before the initiation of tube feeding. If a nasoduodenal or jejunal placement is desired, pass the additional 20 to 30 cm of tubing left extending from the nose transpylorically at a rate of approximately 5 cm/hr. Placing the patient in the right lateral position will facilitate spontaneous peristaltic advancement of the tube feeding. Obtain an abdominal x-ray after 12 to 24 hours in this position. In the ambulatory patient, the tube will pass spontaneously to the small intestine about 50% of the time.
2. Once the gastric location is confirmed, pull the feeding tube back to 30 cm and remove the guide wire.
3. Make a 30 degree bend at the end of the guide wire at 3 cm from the distal tip.
4. Rethread the guide wire. Some sources warn against reinstering the guide wire because it may cause perforation of the feeding tube or exit the tube into the GI tract.
5. Attach 50-ml syringe to the proximal end of the tube to assist in the rotation of the tube during passage, to aspirate gastric contents, and to inject air for auscultation.
6. Advance the tube a few cm at a time while slowly rotating the attached syringe. This causes the distal end to rotate in a circular motion in an attempt to hook the pyloric outlet. Twenty additional centimeters of tube should be passed for duodenal placement and 30 cm for jejunal placement.

7. With experience, practitioners can usually feel the tip hit the stomach wall and bounce slightly. As the tip is rotated, practitioners will be able to feel it pass through the pylorus. The feeding tube will pass out through the pylorus and loop back on itself. When the tube loops back past the pylorus, the practitioner will feel a sudden loss of resistance as the tube is advanced.

8. Once the tube passes the pylorus, a low-grade resistance will be felt as the tube is advanced into the small bowel. If the tube loops back toward the pylorus and resistance is lost, repeat the procedure. It may take 5 to 20 trials.

9. To confirm placement into the small intestine, instill 5 to 20 ml of air and auscultate for sounds or air. At the proximal duodenum the sounds are higher pitched and heard over the right upper quadrant (RUQ) and do not radiate to the left upper quadrant (LUQ). Sounds are transmitted to the LUQ and flank when the tube enters the distal duodenum. Little air can be aspirated from the small bowel as compared to the stomach. The aspiration of bile suggests a postpyloric placement. The duodenal pH is greater than 7 to 8, whereas gastric pH is usually 4 to 5.

10. Confirm the placement with an abdominal x-ray examination.

Feeding instructions

Check residuals before each feeding; hold the feeding if the residuals are greater than 100 to 150 cc for bolus feeding or of a volume that is greater than twice the hourly rate for continuous feeding. For infants or children, calculate the appropriate residual body weight. It may be as small as 3 to 5 cc.

1. Attach the feeding catheter to the feeding bag or syringe.
2. Clamp off the lower portion of the catheter with fingers or a clamp.
3. Fill the syringe or feeding bag with the feeding.
4. Open the safety plug on the button and attach the adapter and feeding catheter to the button.
5. Elevate the feeding above the level of the stomach and allow gravity flow over 15 to 30 minutes.
6. Refill the syringe before it empties to prevent air from reaching the stomach.

7. When the feeding is complete, flush the tube with at least 10 cc tap water.

8. Remove the adapter and feeding tube. No formula should be refluxed because of the reflux valve.

Feeding using a feeding button

1. Determine the depth of the stoma so that the proper size feeding button can be used. At present there are three sizes: small (1.7-cm shaft), medium (2.7-cm shaft), and large (4.3-cm shaft).

2. Once the appropriate size has been chosen distend the button with an abturator to aid in insertion. The obturator should be lubricated with a water-soluble lubricant and the button distended several times before insertion, ensuring the patency of the reflux valve.

3. Lubricate the dome of the button and the stoma with a water-soluble lubricant and introduce it through the gastrostomy site into the stomach.

4. Remove the obturator. The antireflux valve may be sticking to the obturator. If the valve is not properly seated, leakage of gastric contents can occur. Slightly rotating the obturator when removing it may eliminate the problem. If the antireflux valve continues to stick, gently push the obturator back into the button until the valve goes back into its closed position. An 8 or 10 French suction catheter can also be used since it is softer, more flexible, and less likely to damage the stomach than the obturator. Simply insert the catheter until the valve goes back to its closed position.

5. After the obturator or catheter is removed, visually check the position of the antireflux valve to make sure it is closed; then insert the flip-top silicone safety cover. The outer surface of the button should be flush with the skin, and the safety plug remains in place between feedings.

6. The button is radiopaque to allow x-ray exam confirmation of the placement before initiation of feedings.

Postprocedure patient education

Instruct the patient to notify you or the staff if there is migration of the tube or dislodgement, any respiratory difficulty, increased esophageal discomfort, or abdominal discomfort, including cramping, nausea, vomiting, and diarrhea.

Teach the patient to elevate the head of the bed to at least 30 degrees during the feeding.

Checking gastric or intestinal residual is usually not necessary in small-bore tube feedings.

Flush with at least 10 cc water before and after each feeding or medication administration; 30 to 50 cc water is usually recommended.

Clamp the feeding tube when it is not in use.

With continuous feedings, flush every 8 hours.

Instruct the patient to notify you immediately if feeding is discontinued in a patient who is on insulin.

Practitioner Followup/Complications

See Procedure on care of PEGs for management of common problems.

Practitioners monitor the patient's nutritional status with weight and serum chemistry for fluid and electrolyte balance.

Practitioners check the PEG placement by testing pH; gastric pH is acidic at 3; intestinal alkaline at 7.

Practitioners monitor GI tolerance, the status of the feeding tube and site, and for potential adverse nutrient-drug interaction. Frequency for monitoring can be according to the patient's status. For stable patients, monitor every week or more if needed. Monitoring may be reduced for long-term tube feeding but should never be discontinued entirely.

X-ray examination is the only definitive measure to confirm proper placement.

Practitioners assess the patient for abdominal distention, nausea, vomiting, diarrhea, or slowed bowel sounds. Serial abdominal girths can be performed by measuring the girth from one superior iliac crest to another. An increase in 8 to 10 cm above baseline is thought to necessitate the cessation of feedings.

Practitioners also assess for skin breakdown of the nares. Clean the nares with a cotton-tip applicator and peroxide; apply petroleum jelly.

Practitioners evaluate the patient for accidental respiratory placement of the tube by x-ray examination, air insufflation ausculatation, examining aspirate, testing pH, and observing for coughing, cyanosis, or inability to speak. Remove the feeding tube immediately if these are found.

Practitioners should check for esophageal migration. Insufflated air may cause belching in many patients with esophageal placement.

Practitioners monitor for excessive residual. This is often difficult to monitor in small bowel tube placement since it is difficult to aspirate from a small-bore tube. The inference is that it is not necessary to monitor since there is normally little fluid in the small bowel and forward motion is rather rapid. If the patient is intolerant of tube feeding, the practitioner may consider placing a nasogastric tube and measuring the gastric residual. The practitioner should be able to aspirate a small amount of fluid to test for alkaline pH (see Methany and others, 1993).

Practitioners should check for aspiration. Signs of aspiration include decreased mental status, respiratory distress, fever, and agitation. Management of aspiration may include suctioning, arterial blood gases, blood cultures, emergency chest x-ray exam, and antibiotics.

CPT BILLING CODES
91100—Intestinal feeding tube, passage, positioning, and monitoring.

BIBLIOGRAPHY
Bockus S: When your patient needs tube feedings: making the right decisions, *Nursing 93* 23(7):34, 1993.

Cockrell C, Cho S: Placement of enteric feeding tubes using guidewire technique, *Southern Med J* 78(2):210, 1985.

Hull MA, and others: Audit of outcome of long-term enteral nutrition by percutaneous endoscopic gastrostomy, *Lancet* 341(8849):869, 1993.

Huth M, O'Brien M: The gastrostomy feeding tube, *Pediatr Nur* 13(4):24, 1987.

Lysen L: The mechanics of delivery. In Krey SK, Murray RL, editors: *Dynamics of nutritional support: assessment, implementation, evaluation,* Norwalk, Conn, 1986, Appleton-Century-Crofts.

Methany N: Minimizing respiratory complications of nasoenteric tube feedings: state of the science, *Heart & Lung* 22(3):213, 1993.

Methany, N, and others: How to aspirate fluid from small-bore feeding tubes, *Am J Nurs* 93(5):86, 1993.

Perry AG, Potter PA: *Clinical nursing skills and techniques,* ed 3, St Louis, 1994, Mosby.

Varella L: Nasoenteral tube feeding. In Rombeau JL, and others, editors: *Atlas of nutritional support techniques,* Boston, 1989, Little, Brown.

Varella L: Rationale for adult nutrition support guidelines, *J Parenteral Enteral Nutrit* 17(4), 1993.

Zaluga G: Bedside method for placing small bowel feeding tubes in critically ill patients, *Chest* 100(6):1643, 1991.

CHAPTER 7

Musculoskeletal Procedures

Fracture Immobilization

Description

A fracture is a break in the integrity of a bone. The disruption may range from a simple crack to the complete transection of the cortex and medullary canal. Fractures are some of the most common injuries among young, otherwise healthy people. Evaluation of injuries in children requires special consideration. Children's tendons are stronger than their bones. Avulsion and green stick fractures are common, and fractures through the growth plate will not show on x-ray examination. As the age of the general population increases, broken bones are seen more frequently among the elderly as osteopenia and osteoporosis take their toll.

Most fractures presenting to primary care practices are of the "closed" variety, in which the skin overlying the break remains intact. Broken bones themselves are rarely life threatening, but they are frequently associated with injury to nearby supporting joints and to supporting structures such as ligaments and tendons, blood vessels, and nerves.

199

Indications

Primary treatment of fractures most often consists of splinting (and occasionally casting) the known or suspected fracture. After initial stabilization, most fractures should be referred to an orthopedist. Because nondisplaced fractures of either the diaphysis (the middle half of the bone) or the metaphysis (the ossification centers of growing bones) can be difficult to diagnose, any patient with pain (especially pin-point pain), swelling, and ecchymosis over a bony area should be splinted and examined with x-rays. If x-ray examination is available, at a minimum, anterior-posterior and lateral views of the injured extremity should be obtained.

Known or suspected fractures that are displaced and those near articular surfaces should always be referred to an orthopedist for definitive care. In children, fractures involving the growth plate also warrant special attention. Patients should be splinted before their referral out of the primary care office.

Contraindications/Precautions

There are few absolute contraindictions to splinting, but one may be in the case of fracture with severe limb deformity. In these instances, gentle manual traction to straighten the limb may be applied by trained personnel.

Although contraindications to splinting are few, precautions are numerous. The practitioner must be aware that the early complications of fracture include damage to nerves and blood vessels, ligament disruption with associated joint instability, and skin breakdown. Compartment syndrome may occur with any long bone fracture, although it is most common with lower leg trauma.

Unstable fractures may require surgical reduction. Improper splinting may aggravate or induce complications. X-ray films may be taken after the splint has been placed (unless a metal splint is used).

Patient Preparation/Education

Practitioners explain to the patient that splinting and immobilization of the injured area is a temporary intervention to reduce pain and the risk of further damage to adjacent soft tissues. The casting tape will be placed in some water to begin the chemical reaction that will harden the fiberglass. As the splint hardens, it will become warm, but the warmth will be temporary.

Practitioners should instruct the patient that the splint is to remain in place at all times, unless the patient is instructed by a health care professional to remove it.

Equipment

- Casting tape (fiberglass or plaster of paris) or preformed, cut-to-length splinting material
- Synthetic cast padding
- Bandage scissors
- Gloves
- Ace wrap
- Bucket of water

Procedure

1. Using the roll of castpadding, measure out a length long enough to include the joint distal to the injury. The joint proximal to the injury should also be included if feasible (for example, distal radius fractures do not usually need to include the elbow).
2. Layer the padding to make four to six layers. Cut or tear another single layer of padding the same length.
3. Don gloves. Dip the splinting material in the water for 10 to 15 seconds. Gently wipe excess water from the splinting material. Do not wring out the material.
4. Repeat the layering process with fiberglass splinting. The splinting material should also be 4 to 6 layers thick.
5. Place the single layer of padding over the fiberglass to form a "sandwich" of padding-splint-padding.
6. Place the heavily padded side of the splint against the limb and, while maintaining the limb in anatomic alignment, quickly secure the splint with the ace bandage. Do not stretch the ace bandage while wrapping the splint because this may result in neurovascular compromise. The splint will harden and dry in 10 to 15 minutes.

Postprocedure patient education

Inform the patient that the splint is temporary but should not be removed by the patient.

Instruct the patient to notify you if pain significantly worsens or swelling, numbness, coldness, or tingling of the splinted area occurs.

Practitioner Followup/Complications

Patients with a documented fracture should be referred to an orthopedist for definitive care. If x-ray films are unavailable or inconclusive, patients should be referred to an orthopedist within 24 to 48 hours. If the x-ray examination was done in the primary care office, the films should accompany the patient to the orthopedic surgeon.

CPT BILLING CODES

29105—Application of long arm splint (shoulder to hand).

29125—Application of short arm splint (forearm to hand); static.

29126—Application of short arm splint (forearm to hand): dynamic.

29103—Application of finger splint; static.

29131—Application of finger splint: dynamic.

29505—Application of long leg splint (thigh to ankle or toes).

29515—Application of short leg splint (calf to foot).

BIBLIOGRAPHY

Dunwood CJ: Modalities for immobilization. In Maher AB, Salmond SW, Pellino TA, editors: *Orthopaedic nursing,* 278, Philadelphia, 1994, WB Saunders.

Heckman JD: Fractures: emergency care and complications, *Clin Symp* 43(3), 1992.

Splinting—Wrist and Hand

Description

Splinting is a commonly used therapeutic procedure performed in the primary care setting for the management of hand and wrist injuries. Splinting is a temporary or adjunct therapy used to stabilize an injured limb. Although splinting in general does not provide enough support to immobilize forearm or wrist fractures it is an important initial procedure in fracture care.

Indications

Any injury to the wrist or hand that involves torn or stretched tendons or ligaments should be splinted.

Stable fractures should be splinted.

Inflammatory processes such as tenosynovitis (which involves the muscle-tendon complex).

Congenital or acquired deformitis (radial club hand, arthritis).

Conditions requiring temporary immobilization to reduce inflammation (carpal tunnel syndrome, tendinitis).

Contraindications/Precautions

Splinting is a temporary therapy. Improper or inordinately long periods of splinting may result in functional limitation or deformity of the affected area. Some preformed splints are difficult to apply snugly enough to ensure proper fit.

Patient Preparation/Education

Patients should be told the reason for splinting, how their wrist or hand is to be positioned as the splint is applied, when the splint may be removed (if at all) by the patients, the expected duration of splinting, and how to keep the splint clean and dry.

While the splint is being applied, explain that as the splinting material hardens (if it is plaster or fiberglass), it becomes quite warm. The heat given off is temporary and will subside within a few minutes.

Equipment

- Rigid or semirigid material 3 to 4 inches wide (fiberglass or plaster casting tape), padded aluminum splints (for fingers), or preformed splints

- Padding material
- Water
- Nonsterile gloves
- Scissors
- Ace wrap
- Tape (¼-inch adhesive or silk)

Procedure

A. Wrist–Fig. 7-1

1. Inspect the skin for any breaks in integrity; do not splint over major open wounds.
2. Measure the patient's arm from the metacarpophalangeal joints to 1-inch distal to the elbow. Unroll the cast padding to that same length, making 6 to 8 layers. Make one more layer of padding the same length, making 6 to 8 layers. Make one more layer of padding the same length; set it aside.
3. Don gloves. Dip the casting tape in water for 10 to 15 seconds; gently squeeze excess water from tape.
4. Unroll four to six layers of casting tape on top of the layered padding. Place the final single layer of padding on top of the casting tape.
5. With the wrist in the appropriate position (see Fig. 7-3), place the layered padding side of the splint against the skin; secure it with an ace wrap. Do not stretch the ace wrap while securing the splint.
6. One the splint is in place, use the palm of your hand to mold the splint to the patient's wrist and arm. The splint will harden in about 10 minutes.

B. Fingers–Fig. 7-2

Note: When splinting fingers, make every attempt to prevent shortening of the collateral ligaments of the digit. The "safe" position of splinting (Fig. 7-3) maintains the metacarpophalangeal (MCP) joint in 70 degrees of flexion and the proximal interphalangeal (PIP) joint in 20 degrees flexion. The so-called "position of function" used in splint-

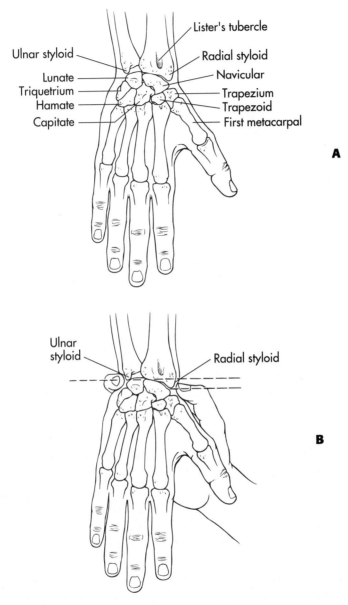

Fig. 7-1 **A** Bones of the wrist (dorsal aspect). **B** Reference points in palpation of the wrist. The radial styloid process is more distal than the ulnar.

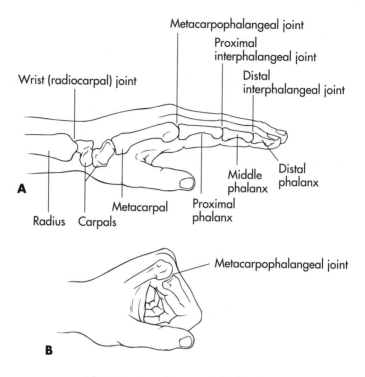

Fig. 7-2 Carpal bones of the hand.

ing finger fractures and sprains may result in loss of hand function secondary to collateral ligament shortening (Fig. 7-3).

1. Before splinting, examine the finger carefully for evidence of rotational deformity. This can be accomplished by having the patient sit opposite the practitioner. The patient then places their palms up and flexes the MCP joints to 90 degrees. The practitioner then examines the digits from the distal end and notes the orientation of the nail beds and distal finger pads. Normally, the nail beds should be in pretty much the same plane.

2. Then instruct the patient to "make a fist" while keeping the PIP and distal interphalangeal (DIP) joints straight; if there is over- or underriding of a digit that is different from the contralateral hand, there is evidence of rotational deformity. Refer these patients immediately to a hand specialist or orthopedist.

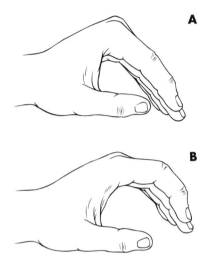

Fig. 7-3 Positions of hand immobilization. **A** "Safe position" (James). **B** "Position of function."

3. Using the contralateral uninjured digit as a template, measure from the tip of the finger to the heel of the hand.
4. Using scissors, cut a padded aluminum splint to this length. Splints may be applied to either the dorsal or the volar surface of the digit; if in doubt, the volar surface is generally safe.
5. Again using the contralateral digit as a guide, place the digit in the "safe" position.
6. Once the splint is appropriately bent, attach it to the injured finger with ¼-inch tape. If additional security is necessary, "buddy tape" the splinted digit to the adjacent digit.

Postprocedure patient education

Educate the patients about signs of neurovascular compromise and/or pressure areas.

Instruct the patients that they may loosen the ace wrap if throbbing, pain, or swelling increase.

Instruct the patients to contact the primary care practitioner if loosening the ace wrap and elevating the wrist do not relieve symptoms.

Practitioner Followup/Complications

Followup should be determined by the type and severity of the injury. The patient with a known or suspected fracture should be referred to an orthopedist within 1 to 2 days of the injury.

Complications of improper splinting include skin breakdown beneath the splint, contracture, and functional deficit. Flexor or extensor tendon tears of the fingers that are improperly or inadequately splinted may result in a permanent loss of function.

Tendon injuries must be immediately referred to an orthopedist or hand specialist.

CPT BILLING CODES

26600—Closed treatment of metacarpal fracture, single; each bone.

26750—Closed treatment of distal phalangeal fracture, finger or thumb: without manipulation, each bone.

25622—Closed treatment of carpal scaphoid (navicular) fracture, with or without internal or external fixation.

25630—Closed treatment of carpal bone fracture, excluding navicula; without manipulation, each bone.

25650—Closed treatment of ulnar styloid fracture.

25500—Closed treatment of radial shaft fracture; without manipulation.

25530—Closed treatment of ulnar shaft fracture; without manipulation.

25600—Closed treatment of distal radial fracture (e.g., Colles or Smith type) or epiphyseal separation, with or without fracture of ulnar styloid; without manipulation.

BIBLIOGRAPHY

Caillet R: *Hand pain and impairment,* ed 2, Philadelphia, 1975, FA Davis.
Gates SJ, Mooar PA, editors: *Orthopaedic and sports medicine for nurses: common problems in management,* Baltimore, 1989, Williams & Wilkins.
Green DP, editor: *Operative hand surgery,* ed 2, New York, 1988, Churchill Livingstone.
Hilt NE, Cogburn SB: *Manual of orthopedics,* St Louis, 1980, Mosby.
Mercier LR: *Practical orthopedics,* ed 3, St Louis, 1991, Mosby.
Reilly BM: *Practical strategies in outpatient medicine,* ed 2, Philadelphia, 1991, WB Saunders.
Tinker RV, editor: *Orthopaedics in primary care,* Baltimore, 1984, Williams & Wilkins.
Winspur I: Emergency care of the injured and: hand dressings, splints and casts, *Emerg Med Services* January/February, 22, 1980.

Splinting—Ankle Sprains

Description

Sprains are the most common injury to the ankle seen in the emergency department or by the primary care practitioner. "Simple sprains," although common, are frequently inappropriately treated, because many practitioners have a limited understanding of ankle anatomy and physiology. Proper assessment and treatment of ankle injuries is essential to promoting return of motion and function.

An ankle sprain is any stretching or tearing of the lateral or medial ligaments surrounding the joint as the result of excessive force being applied by inversion, eversion, or hyperextension. Inversion injuries to the ankle are most common. Ankle injuries occur in every age population but are more prevalent in childhood through late middle age.

The ankle joint is primarily stabilized by two sets of ligaments: the lateral collateral ligaments (made up of the anterior talofibular, calcaneofibular, and the posterior talofibular ligaments) and the medial or deltoid ligaments. The most commonly injured ligament of the ankle is the anterior talofibular ligament; this occurs when an inversion stress is applied. The calcaneofibular ligament joins the so-called upper and lower ankle joints; this is the second most commonly injured ligament. The posterior talofibular ligament is the strongest of the three and is least likely to be injured in a common malleolar sprain (Fig. 7-4, *A*).

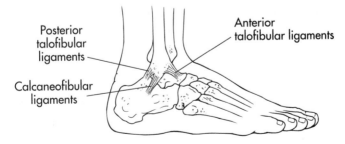

Posterior
talofibular
ligaments

Calcaneofibular
ligaments

Anterior
talofibular ligaments

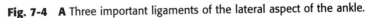

Fig. 7-4   A Three important ligaments of the lateral aspect of the ankle.

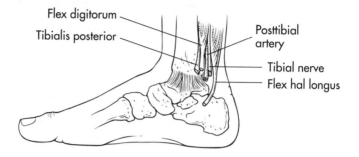

Fig. 7-4 **B** Deltoid ligament.

Eversion injuries, which result in damage to the medial malleolus, are much less common than inversion injuries. The deltoid ligament is the broadest and thickest ligament in the ankle; therefore, it is more difficult to sustain excessive stress to this ligament. Medial malleolar sprains may result in an avulsion of the distal medial tip of the tibia (the medial malleolus). As force is continued in an eversion injury, the inferior tibiofibular ligament and interosseous membrane may tear (Fig. 7-4, *B*).

Indications

Ankle sprains are classified into three grades, based on pathology, function, and instability (Table 7-1).

Grade I injuries are those resulting from minor stretching without tearing of the involved ligament or ligaments and have no joint instability.

Grade II sprains consist of partial tearing of the involved ligaments with some joint instability. This is a moderate injury which results in some compromise of function.

Grade III injuries are marked by significant swelling, ecchymosis, and instability of the joint. These are the result of a complete tear of the ligament.

Patients presenting with signs of grade III sprains should be referred to an orthopedic surgeon. Some grade I sprains may be treated by the primary care practitioner, but it is more prudent to refer these patients as well.

Table 7-1

Clinical Diagnosis of Ligament Injury

	First-degree sprain	Second-degree sprain	Third-degree sprain
Synonym	Mild sprain	Moderate sprain	Severe sprain
Etiology	Direct or indirect trauma to joint	Same	Severe direct or indirect trauma to joint
Symptoms	Pain; mild disability	Pain; moderate disability	Pain; severe disability
Signs	Mild point tenderness; no abnormal motion; little or no swelling	Point tenderness; moderate loss of function; slight to moderate abnormal motion; swelling; localized hemorrhage	Loss of function; marked abnormal motion; possible deformity; x-rays: stress films demonstrate abnormal motion
Complications	Tendency to recurrence; aggravation	Tendency to recurrence, aggravation; persistent instability; traumatic arthritis	Persistent instability; traumatic arthritis
Pathology	Minor tearing of ligament	Partial tear of ligament	Complete tear of ligament

Source: *Standard Nomenclature of Athletic Injuries,* American Medical Association, Chicago, 1976.
From: American Academy of Orthopaedic Surgeons: (1991) *Athletic Training and Sports Medicine,* 2nd ed., Park Ridge, Ill, 1991, American Academy of Orthopaedic Surgeons, p. 413.

Specific Tests

Anterior drawer test (Fig. 7-5): This test is used to increase stress on the anterior talofibular ligament. If straight anterior movement of the talus occurs, it indicates both medial and lateral ligament insufficiency. If only one side moves forward, there is ipsilateral insufficiency.

Talar tilt test (Fig. 7-6): This test is used to determine whether the calcaneofibular ligament is torn. The patient lies on his or her side while the examiner holds the foot in anatomic alignment with the leg parallel to the floor. The talus is then tilted from side to side. The calcaneofibular ligament is stressed when the foot is tilted into adduction.

Thompson test (Fig. 7-7): This test measures the integrity of the Achilles' tendon. The patient kneels on a chair with his feet hanging over the front of the seat. The practitioner compresses the calf muscles; if there is no plantar flexion of the foot, the test is positive for Achilles' tendon rupture.

Radiographic examination: Ideally three views of the ankle should be taken in order to rule out fracture or dislocation.

AP view: Anterior-posterior viewing allows for examination of the joint space and any obvious fracture of the distal tibia or fibula should be visible. An AP view also allows evaluation of the talus.

Lateral view: A lateral viewing allows better view of talus, calcaneus; it is easier to see a spiral fracture of the distal fibula.

Mortise view: A mortise view is similar to the AP view but the foot and ankle are rotated 15 to 30 degrees. This view is best for evaluating the ankle mortise.

Contraindications/Precautions

Careful evaluation of the ankle must be made before any splinting. Any ankle instability should be referred to an orthopedist.

Fractures of the foot (proximal fifth metatarsal), syndesmosis rupture, Achilles' tendon rupture, infection (osteomyelitis, septic joint), osteochronditis dessicans of the talus, and tumor are all possible other etiologies for ankle pain and swelling.

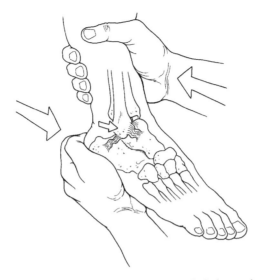

Fig. 7-5 The calcaneus (and talus) move anteriorly beneath the tibia when there is ligamentous disruption of the ankle joint. This is a positive "anterior drawer" sign.

Knowledge of a few special tests is important to diagnose the severity of injury accurately. Once properly evaluated, ankle sprains can be appropriately treated. For specific evaluation tests see the box.

Patient Preparation/Education

Patients should be informed about the purpose of splinting and its expected duration.

Practitioners explain to the patient that splinting and immobilization of the injured area is a temporary intervention to reduce pain and the risk of further damage to adjacent soft tissues.

Practitioners should describe the casting procedure by explaining that the casting tape will be placed in some water to begin the chemical reaction that will harden the fiberglass. As the splint hardens, it will become warm, but the warmth will be temporary.

The splint is to remain in place at all times, unless the patient is instructed by a health care professional to remove it.

Practitioners reassure the patient that this procedure should not hurt. A sprain often is as painful as a fracture, and this immobilization will actually lessen pain overall.

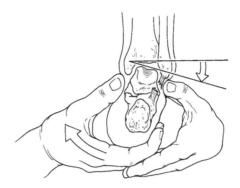

Fig. 7-6 If both the anterior talofibular and calcaneofibular ligaments are disrupted, the ankle is unstable on "talar tilt" testing.

Practitioners should reinforce that splinting will require the patient's cooperation in holding the proper position. It may take some time to complete the proper splinting procedure.

Equipment

The initial treatment of ankle injuries (first 24 to 48 hours) consists of RICE—rest, ice, compression, and evaluation. The RICE regimen limits soft tissue swelling and helps reduce the risk of further injury. Ice also helps as a local anesthetic and may relieve some muscle spasm.

- Ice bag or chemical cold pack
- Ankle immobilizer (aircast or other)
- Splinting or casting material
- Cast padding, water, gloves
- Scissors
- Ace bandages

Procedure

Ace bandages alone are insufficient support for anything but a grade I sprain. Significant ankle sprains require support strong enough to prevent movement of the joint.

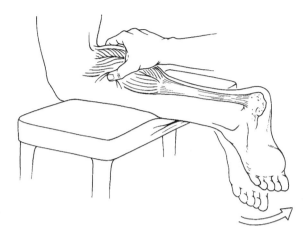

Fig. 7-7 Squeezing the muscles in the calf should elicit plantar flexion of the foot when the Achilles' tendon is intact. This Thompson test is most useful when there is prominent heel and calf pain and pain prevents adequate examination of the Achilles' apparatus. A negative (normal) Thompson test in this case provides reassurance that the Achilles' tendon is not ruptured.

Aircast splint:

1. Inflate the air bags.
2. Apply the rigid medial and lateral supports to the ankle.
3. Once the side pieces are in place, secure the heel strap (the rounded edge of the calcaneal strap follows the contour of the heel).
4. Fasten the Velcro straps.

Splint:

1. Have the patient lie prone on a table with the injured leg flexed to 90 degrees at the knee. This assists in maintaining a 90 degree angle at the ankle.
2. Measure a length of cast padding along the posterior lower leg, from the tip of the toes to just below the knee.
3. Unroll several layers of padding this same length (or wrap the foot and lower leg with padding).
4. Using the first measured length of padding as a guide, wet and unroll six to eight layers of casting tape to the same length.
5. Place the casting layers on the posterior leg and the entire bottom of foot.
6. Secure with an ace wrap.

Postprocedure patient education

Teach patients how and when to use ice, compression, elevation, moist heat, crutches, and physical therapy.

Cryotherapy: Apply an ice pack to the joint for 10- to 20-minute periods tid or qid. Ice should generally be discontinued after the first 24 to 48 hours postinjury. A compressive dressing such as an ace wrap may also reduce swelling if the ankle is not splinted.

Crutches: Crutches may be used for the first several days to avoid placing additional stress on an already damaged joint.

Teach patients a three-point gait wherein both crutches and the nonsupportive leg go forward, then the good leg comes through. The crutches are immediately brought forward and the pattern is repeated.

Proper sizing of the crutches to the patient is crucial to successful crutch walking. To ensure proper placement, place the crutch tips 6 to 8 inches from the side of each foot (using a short forward placement of the crutches to maximize stability), and measure the upper pads for fit. They should be 2 or 3 finger breadths below the axilla, with the elbows slightly bent.

Moist heat: Moist heat, such as hot, wet towels, soaking the ankle in warm water, or using a moist heating pad for 10 to 20 minutes bid will improve circulation and ease some of the stiffness associated with ligamentous tearing.

Physical therapy: Physical therapy is begun as soon as painfree exercise is possible, usually within 1 to 2 weeks of injury. Exercises begin with range of motion and then isometric, isotonic, and isokinetic activities for dorsiflexion, plantar flexion, inversion, and eversion. Athletes and the elderly should be directed to a formal physical therapy program, whereas many otherwise healthy, motivated people may use a home exercise program.

Make sure the patient can reiterate the signs and symptoms of neurovascular impairment: tingling, numbness, blanching of skin.

Pain control may be achieved through use of common nonsteroidal antiinflammatory medications (NSAIDs), with high doses at regular intervals often required. Patients on NSAID therapy should be aware of the purpose, dosage, side effects, and toxicities of their particular medication.

Inform patients that ankle sprains may take some time to heal. Even after 6 to 8 weeks of healing, there may be residual problems such as increased joint size and increased sensitivity to barometric pressure changes.

Practitioner Followup/Complications

Complications of ankle sprain include ankle instability and weakness; surgical repair for this is still controversial.

Recurrent sprains are associated with inadequate immobilization for sufficient time while ligamentous healing occurs. Recurrent swelling is fairly common and may persist for many months.

Patients are generally followed from 2 to 4 weeks, as needed. If symptoms of pain or joint instability persist on followup, the patient should be referred to an orthopedist.

CPT BILLING CODES

99202—Initial office visit, low complexity (such as simple sprain).

99203—Initial office visit, moderate complexity (such as sports injury).

29540—Strapping of ankle.

29515—Application of short leg splint (calf to foot).

BIBLIOGRAPHY

American Academy of Orthopaedic Surgeons: *Athletic training and sports medicine,* ed 2, Park Ridge, Ill, 1991, American Academy of Orthopaedic Surgeons.

Barker LR, Burton JR, Zieve PD: *Principles of ambulatory medicine,* ed 2, Baltimore, 1986, Williams & Wilkins, p. 883.

Dvorkin ML: *Office orthopaedics,* Norwalk, Conn, 1993, Appleton & Lange, p. 240.

Kimura I, Nawoczenski D, and Mulley AG: Effect of the air stirrup in controlling ankle inversion stress, *J Orthoped Sports Phys Ther,* 9:190, 1987.

Magee DJ: *Orthopedic Physical Assessment,* Philadelphia, 1992, WB Saunders, p. 448.

Sammarco G: *Foot and ankle manual,* Philadelphia, 1991, Lea & Febiger.

Simon R, Koenigsknecht S: *Orthopaedic emergency medicine: the extremities,* New York, 1982, Appleton.

Stover CN: Functional sprain management of the ankle, *Ambul Care,* 6:25, 1986.

Reduction of Subluxed Radial Head

Description

A subluxed radial head is a tear in the distal attachment of the annular ligament through which the radial head protrudes. The proximal portion of the annular ligament slips into the radio-humeral joint. This injury occurs in children 1 to 5 years of age, with about 50% presenting with severe pain and inability to move the arm following a sudden pull on the child's hand. the child may also report feeling a click.

Indication

Listen for a history consistent with a subluxed radial head. The child often presents carrying the injured arm limply against the body, or supported with the other hand. The forearm is usually pronated with the elbow slightly flexed. Tenderness may be palpated over the anterolateral aspect of the radial head. Passive flexion and extension of the elbow is tolerated within a 30 to 120 degree range. The child strongly resists passive supination of the forearm. The exam of the shoulder, wrist, and clavicle are unremarkable.

Contraindications/Precautions

If swelling, ecchymosis, or other injury is noted, refer the patient to an orthopedic specialist.

Patient Preparation/Education

Practitioners outline the steps of the procedure.
Practitioners should explain how long this will take.
Practitioners should warn the child that there will be momentary discomfort.

Procedure

1. Support the elbow with your hand and place your thumb over the radial head.
2. Supinate or pronate the forearm in one fast motion. A click should be felt and may even be heard. This signals the reduction has taken place.
3. The child should begin to use his or her arm with full range of motion within 30 minutes. No sling or restraint is necessary.

Postprocedure patient education

Instruct the patient to return for followup within 1 week.

Educate parents against pulling on the child's hand.

Instruct parents to watch for signs of restricted arm use occurring or a repeated subluxation.

Instruct the patient's parents to seek medical attention if fever, erythema, or edema occur around joint.

Practitioner Followup/Complications

If the practitioner does not feel a click the reduction is probably not complete.

Failure to achieve or maintain reduction is more frequent in injuries less than 2 hours old.

If full range on motion is not achieved, have the child wait 2 hours, then repeat procedure.

Five percent of children will have recurrences. Refer to an orthopedic specialist.

CPT BILLING CODES

94640—Closed treatment of radial head subluxation in child, "nursemaid elbow," with manipulation.

BIBLIOGRAPHY

Frumkin K: Nursemaid's elbow: a radiographic demonstration, *Ann Emerg Med* 14(7): 690, 1985.

Nichols HH: Nursemaid's elbow: reducing it to simple terms, *Contemp Pediatr* 5(5):50, 1988.

Quan L, Marcuse E: The epidemiology and treatment of radial head subluxation, *Am J Dis Children* 139:1194, 1985.

CHAPTER 8

Metabolic/Miscellaneous Procedures

X-ray Interpretation

Description

X-ray examinations are used in a variety of clinical settings to confirm clinical impressions. Depending on the power setting, x-rays penetrate body tissues to varying degrees. As such, they are useful in evaluating some internal soft tissue as well as bones. Although the nurse practitioner should have a basic knowledge of x-ray film interpretation, a definitive reading must be done by a qualified physician.

Indications

Radiographic evaluation of a patient should be done whenever there is clinical suspicion of pulmonary disease, intraabdominal air fluid levels, abdominal aortic aneurysm, and bone or joint abnormalities.

Contraindications/Precautions

Caution should be used when obtaining x-rays films (plain films) as the generally easy accessibility to other diagnostic tools such as

221

computerized tomography (CT) may make other tests more appropriate. There are few contraindications to ordering and interpreting x-ray films. However, it should be kept in mind that children, men, and women of reproductive age, and especially women in the first trimester of pregnancy should have their gonads shielded. Unless an x-ray examination is essential to diagnosis and treatment of a pregnant patient, it should be deferred.

Procedure

When interpreting x-ray films, develop a logical system and follow that system consistently. Two sample systems follow.

Chest x-ray exam

1. *Overall appearance:* Both lung fields should be equally illuminated. The background of the film should be black. Unexposed areas such as the heart should be white to blue white in color.
2. *Diaphragm:* Note its level and shape (curved, elevated, flattened). Is there evidence of air in the subdiaphragmatic space?
3. *Heart:* Examine its size, shape, and location.
4. *Trachea:* Its position should be midline; its width should be fairly even.
5. *Hila:* The hila normally have a butterfly-like appearance. The right side is usually slightly lower than the left.
6. *Mediastinum:* Examine the blood vessels (a normal width ratio with the rest of the chest cavity width should be no more than 1:3). Look for the presence of air.
7. *Lung fields:* These should be equally lucent without opacities, cysts, or air/fluid levels. Bronchi are NOT normally distinctly visible. Peripheral lung fields should be easily seen.
8. *Skeletal structures:* Look for rotation of vertebrae (normally, posterior spinous processes will line up in the same plane). Trace ribs out to lateral edges; some fractures can be quite subtle.
9. *Evaluate shadows.* Define the position of breasts and nipples in women, nipples in men. Overlying neck muscles may cloud the apices of both lungs.

Bony films

1. *Overall size and shape of bone:* Look for extra calcification, abnormal contour.
2. *Local size and shape of bone:* Keep the patient's age in mind. Is there appropriate skeletal maturity? Are epiphyseal growth plates open or closed?
3. *Cortex:* Look at thickness, contour, and integrity. Normal adult cortex thins with age. At any age, a lytic lesion involving more than 50% of the cortex is an indication for surgery and/or prophylactic fixation.
4. *Trabecular pattern:* This is more easily visible in larger bones (iliac crest, greater trochanter, femoral neck). Look for unusual density or lucency, tumor.
5. *Bone density:* The density of the entire bone should be pretty much consistent. Before changes become apparent 30% to 35% of bone mass must be lost. With local density changes look for evidence of fracture (new or healed), tumor, sclerosis.
6. *Margins of local lesions:* Are there calcifications in surrounding tissue? Do lesions invade the medullary canal or surrounding soft tissue? Chronic osteomyelitis may show bone and soft tissue inflammation.
7. *Bone continuity:* Look for fracture lines or displacement of fracture fragments. Look at the symmetry of the joint lines. For example, no more than 2 mm of difference between the joint spaces should be present in an intact ankle mortise.
8. *Periosteal change:* Periosteal thickening may be the only objective initial evidence of stress fracture or acute inflammatory process. Chronic osteomyelitis will show changes in soft tissues overlying infected bone.

Interpretation of results

Abnormalities should be reviewed by a qualified physician to differentiate pathology from normal variants.

Postprocedure patient education

X-ray examinations may need to be repeated after a reasonable length of appropriate treatment. Pulmonary infections may require followup in 1 to 2 weeks to document resolution of infiltrates. Fractures should be reevaluated once immobilization has been discontinued.

BIBLIOGRAPHY

Magee DJ: *Orthopedic physical assessment,* ed 2, Philadelphia, 1992, W. B. Saunders.
Netter FH: *Infection in the Ciba collection of medical illustrations,* vol 8, *Musculoskeletal system, part III: trauma, evaluation and management,* Summit, NJ, 1993, Ciba-Geigy.
Reider B: *Sports medicine: the school-age athlete,* Philadelphia, 1991, W. B. Saunders.

Finger Stick Blood Glucose

Description

Finger stick blood glucose is a method of measuring blood glucose levels using a fingertip drop of blood. Using this technique, diabetic patients can monitor their own glucose levels while at home. Blood glucose monitoring can be done by using either a blood glucose meter or a visual strip. Monitoring blood glucose levels regularly makes it easier to keep blood sugar levels in a normal range. Maintenance of a normal glucose can help reduce health complications that have been linked to diabetes. The self-monitoring blood glucose results can help the patient and the health care provider with planning meals, medication, and exercise regimens.

Indications

Finger stick blood glucose monitoring is indicated for

- Regulation of insulin
- Screening for hypoglycemia and hyperglycemia
- Confirmation of symptomatic glycemic reactions
- Monitoring blood sugar in pregnant diabetics

- Helping control blood sugar in clients with unstable diabetes or those using an insulin infusion pump
- Monitoring blood sugar in clients with newly diagnosed diabetes

Contraindications/Precautions

Practitioners follow universal blood and body fluid precautions. Practitioners use aseptic technique.

The finger stick blood glucose technique should not be used if one of the following conditions apply:

- Vision deterioration or color blindness
- Patients are physically and mentally handicapped and cannot perform the procedure
- Severe vasoconstrictive diseases, such as, Raynaud's disease
- Patients considered for monitoring should not have severe anemia or polycythemia because the values obtained for blood glucose may be markedly affected by these conditions. Anemia falsely elevates and polycythemia falsely depresses blood glucose values. Hematocrit values between 30% and 55% have no affect on the test results.

The instructions that accompany the particular brand of equipment should be followed.

Patient Preparation/Education

Patients need to learn when to test (which depends on the individual patient). Tests should be made ½ hour before meals and at bedtime, whenever the patient feels ill or has signs of hypoglycemia or hyperglycemia, after vigorous exercise, 2 hours after eating, and whenever there has been increased stress or anxiety.

Equipment

- Test strip
- Alcohol swab
- Lancet

- Finger sticking device (optional)
- Cotton ball
- Watch with second hand (not needed with monitor)
- Calibrated monitor
- Disposable gloves
- Paper towel to work on

Procedure

A. Prepare the machine.

1. Check the expiration date on the testing strips; do not use out-dated strips.
2. Remove the test strip from its container immediately before the procedure and recap the container immediately.
3. Calibrate the monitor periodically, following the instructions for the particular machine.

B. Obtain a drop of blood.

1. Hold the patient's arm downward for at least 30 seconds.
2. Clean the selected fingertip with an alcohol swab. Allow the alcohol to dry completely.
3. Prick the finger with the lancet. Stick the side of the finger, and not the fleshy center pad, to avoid painful fingertips. Rotate the finger site sticks to prevent making fingertips sore.
4. Hold the pricked finger, with the hand palm down, and squeeze it firmly until a large handling drop of welled-up blood has formed.
5. Bring the strip to the finger and transfer the blood by lightly touching the reagent area of the strip to the drop. Be sure to cover the reagent area completely; do not smear. Simultaneously, start timing.

C. Follow the steps for the particular brand:

1. Using the Chemstrip bG blood glucose test strip test vial
   a. Wait exactly 60 seconds.
   b. Using moderate pressure, wipe off the blood with one clean,

dry cotton ball. Lightly wipe the strip two more times using the clean sides of the cotton ball. (Important: All blood and cotton residue must be wiped from the test area.)

c. Wait one additional minute.

d. Match the two colors of the reagent area to the color blocks on the vial label. If the two colors on the reagent strip match one of the color blocks, then the value of that specimen is close to the stated value for that block. (For example, if both the top and bottom colors on the strip match the top and bottom colors on the 80 mg/dl color block, then the blood glucose value can be stated as being 80 mg/dl.)

At times the closest match may be one reagent pad corresponding to one blood glucose concentration, and the other pad corresponding to the next higher (or lower) value. In such cases, the blood glucose can be estimated to be about in the middle of these two values. For example, if the blue pad matches the bottom blue of 180 mg/dl and the green pad matches the top green color corresponding to 240 mg/dl, the blood glucose concentration can be considered to around 210 mg/dl.

NOTE: If the color values on the strip are approximately 240 mg/dl or more, wait one more minute for a final reading. The color reaction at 2 minutes (less than 240 mg/dl) and 3 minutes (over 240 mg/dl) are end points and will be stable when stored under proper conditions (protected from direct sunlight, heat, and excessive humidity.) Strips can be dated, saved, and submitted weekly by patients, if the practitioner so desires.

2. Using a blood glucose monitor—Accu-Chek II

   a. After 60 seconds, gently but thoroughly wipe the blood from the test strip with a cotton or rayon ball.

   b. With the timer still running, insert test strip into the meter.

   c. At the end of the second 60-second interval, the blood glucose reading will appear in mg/dl.

3. Using the One Touch II blood glucose monitor

   a. Press the on/off button.

   b. Match the code numbers.

   c. Press the C button until the code number on the meter matches the code number on your current test strip package.

d. Insert the test strip.
e. While insert strip is on display, obtain the blood sample.
f. Apply the blood sample to the test spot. The test strip must be in the meter when you apply the blood. The blood should form a round, shiny drop and completely cover the test spot.
g. Check to make sure the meter is still on.
h. The result appears in 45 seconds.
i. After the result is noted, remove the test strip.

Postprocedure patient education

Be sure each patient is familiar with the owner's booklet and product insert for complete operating instructions and other important information about the machine.

Tell the patient to follow the manufacturer's instructions regarding calibration, testing, and cleaning the machine.

Instruct the patient to keep a log with date, time, and blood glucose level and to bring this log to the practitioner every visit.

Emphasize when to test: During initial intensive monitoring, patients should test 1 hour before and after breakfast, lunch, and dinner and before bedtime. When a pattern of normalization is achieved, patients should test 2 to 4 times daily (patients who monitor fewer than 4 times daily are unlikely to maintain normalization of blood glucose).

Educate the patient regarding possible errors:

If the patient's hands aren't thoroughly washed and dried, false readings can result. If the patient's hands have something sweet and sticky on them, too high a value will result.

Patients sometimes apply too little blood to the strip, causing falsely low readings.

Patients sometimes time the reaction improperly, waiting too long before wiping.

Applying too much pressure when wiping can distort readings.

Inserting the strip incorrectly—with the pads facing away from the on/off button—can create false readings.

Interpretation of results

Ranges of blood glucose that indicate normoglycemia are:

Fasting: 70 to 120 mg/dl
1 to 2 hrs postprandial: less than 140 mg/dl
Nocturnal: not below 50 mg/dl

These are only references; each patient will have his or her own "normal range" that has been decided by the health care provider.

Practitioner Followup/Complications

If blood sugar readings are not consistent with the patient's clinical picture, the machine should be checked before the patient's medications are changed.

The Chemstrip bG reagent strip is designed only for use with fresh whole blood. Use of serum or plasma will register 10% to 15% higher than whole blood.

Adults in a fasting state have arterial and capillary glucose concentrations approximately 5 mg/dl higher than venous blood. In children, the difference may be even greater.

Chemstrip bG reagent strips are based on a glucose oxidase/peroxidase reaction that may have lot-to-lot variations.

Anemia falsely elevates the glucose reading obtained using the Chemstrip bG reagent strip, and polycythemia falsely lowers the blood glucose value. (Hematocrit's between 30% and 55% have no effect on the results).

Chemstrips must always be recapped with the original cap, which contains a drying agent. Do not use the Chemstrip past the expiration date listed on the container. They should also be stored in temperatures above 30°C. The cap should be on the container when it is not in use because the strips deteriorate with exposure to heat, light, and moisture.

Strips of one container should not be compared to the color chart of another container. The color development observed is specific to the container it is packaged in.

BIBLIOGRAPHY

American Diabetes Association: 1-800-232-3472.
Managing your diabetes—a patient guide, Indianapolis, In 46285, Eli Lilly, (317) 276-2950, 1989.
Burritt MF, and others: Portable blood glucose meters, *Postgrad Med* 89(4):75, 1991.

Clinical practice guidelines for treatment of diabetes mellitus. *Canad Med Assoc J* 148 (4):488, 1993.

Guthrie RA: New approaches to improve diabetes control, *Am Fam Physician* 43(2):570, 1991.

Walker EA: Quality assurance for blood glucose monitoring, *Nurs Clin North Am* 28(1):61, 1993.

Bedside Cystometrogram

Description

The bedside cystometrogram is a procedure utilized in gaining information to identify the etiology of urinary incontinence. Although urinary incontinence affects primarily the elderly, it also affects a significant number of younger individuals, especially women. There are four basic types of urinary incontinence: Functional, Overflow, Urge, and Stress.

In addition, there is often overlap between two types of incontinence, for example, urge and stress. This is called mixed incontinence.

Functional incontinence is urinary incontinence, in the presence of a normal functioning urinary tract, that is caused by such factors as immobility, severe cognitive impairment, physical restraints, and medications such as sedatives and antipsychotics. Overflow incontinence is manifested by urinary retention, urinary frequency for small amounts, and much nocturia. It results from an anatomic or physiologic blockage or decreased bladder tone. This can occur with stool impaction, large cystoceles, prostatic hypertrophy, neurologic disorders such as multiple sclerosis and peripheral neuropathy, and medications such as alpha sympathetic agonists, direct smooth muscle relaxants, and all medications having anticholinergic side effects.

Urge incontinence is manifested by an urge to micturate resulting from abnormal bladder contractions and the inability to get to the toilet in time. This can occur with bladder irritants such as infection and inflammation, as with chronic cystitis, estrogen deprivation, increased intraabdominal pressure, structural deformities of the lower urinary tract, and bladder outlet obstruction due to either an anatomic or a neurologic etiology.

Stress incontinence is caused by a problem with urinary outflow control that usually involves the rhabdosphincter and its position relative to the pelvic floor. It is manifested by involuntary urine loss with increased intraabdominal pressure and little nocturia. It affects primarily postmenopausal women with a history of multiple childbirths but it may occur with injury to the bladder muscle after surgery, irradiation, or trauma.

The bladder wall is composed primarily of smooth muscle tissue called the detrusor muscle, which contracts and expels the urine. Abnormal contraction of this muscle is termed *detrusor instability* or *detrusor hyperactivity*. Detrusor instability can be defined as the occurrence of involuntary detrusor contractions greater than or equal to 15 cm of water pressure that occur spontaneously or after provocation while the patient is attempting to inhibit micturition.

Detrusor instability is one of the most common findings among elderly men and women. Although a mixture of stress and urge incontinence is the most common type of incontinence among women, it is estimated that 35% of incontinent women presenting for medical treatment have detrusor instability. Pure stress incontinence occurs in about 27% of women. Urge incontinence is the most common type of incontinence in males and the elderly.

The following are considered necessary for the basic evaluation of urinary incontinence: a comprehensive history, including questioning about urinary symptoms and bowel habits, neurologic symptoms, medications; past medical and surgical conditions, especially those involving the pelvis or urinary system; mental status evaluation; and evaluation for any mobility impairments such as foot problems, general weakness, or disequilibrium. In addition, it can help in the differential diagnosis if the clinician notes the pattern, timing, and amount of urinary incontinence. This can best be evaluated through use of a voiding diary, where the patient records the time and amount of the void, when incontinence occurred, and any comments.

An abdominal, pelvic, rectal, and neurologic examination must also be performed in all patients, with particular attention to saddle sensation and rectal tone. Basic lab work includes a serum BUN and creatinine and a urine culture and urinalysis. If excessive urinary output is detected, however, the basic lab work should include a chemistry panel.

In addition, when evaluating incontinence, practitioners should (1) determine if it is of recent onset (where is it much more likely to be of transient nature and resolve with the resolution of the underlying etiology, e.g., urinary tract infection); (2) identify any risk factors that may be contributing to the incontinence (e.g., an indwelling urinary catheter; (3) identify those potentially serious underlying conditions that may be contributing; (4) utilize the simple urinary incontinence screening procedures available to help differentiate between the types of urinary incontinence and choose appropriate treatment modalities. This can avoid inappropriate treatment and worsening of the urinary incontinence. Practitioners refer patients for further diagnostic urodynamic testing when appropriate (see the guide in the Procedure box).

The bedside cystometrogram measures changes in the bladder pressure in response to filling. Bedside cystometry can provide the clinician with information on the bladder capacity and the postvoid residual volume, detect detrusor stability, and provide an opportunity to perform a stress test at a known volume. It is particularly useful in differentiating between cough-induced detrusor instability and genuine stress incontinence. It has an estimated sensitivity of 75% and a specificity of 79% for detrusor instability, which can be enhanced by standing and repeated testing and provocative maneuvers (e.g., coughing and heel bouncing). A limitation to the use of simple cystometry is its inability to differentiate between bladder pressure increases due to uninhibited bladder contractions and those due to increased intraabdominal pressure.

Indications

Bedside or simple cystometry is indicated for the evaluation of urinary incontinence that is not of a transient or functional nature and that does not resolve when the underlying condition is treated. It is a quick, simple, inexpensive, and fairly reliable test for the diagnosis of detrusor instability and, combined with stress maneuvers, can help to diagnose stress incontinence. In addition, the initial postvoid residual determination can diagnose overflow incontinence cases.

Contraindications/Precautions

Cystometry should not be used in the presence of:

- Current urinary tract infection
- A patient's inability to fully insert the urinary catheter.
- Severe dementia affecting the patient's ability to comprehend or cooperate with the procedure.

Patient Preparation/Education

In preparation for simple cystometry, practitioners obtain a urine specimen for culture and urinalysis and a blood sample for serum BUN and creatinine. Practitioners take a comprehensive history of urinary symptoms and pattern, bowel habits, neurologic symptoms, medications, and past medical and surgical history, and identify all risk factors and potentially serious underlying conditions that may be contributing to the urinary incontinence. Practitioners perform a physical exam that includes abdominal, pelvic, rectal, and neurologic assessments and a mental status evaluation.

The test purpose and basic procedure should be explained to the patient as follows: This test is to determine the cause of urinary incontinence so that appropriate treatment can begin. It involves urinating into a measuring hat, both before and after urinary catheterization; draining the bladder by catheter first, and then filling the bladder with sterile water; and coughing during sitting and standing to observe for urinary incontinence. The procedure takes about 15 to 20 minutes and is associated with minimal, transient discomfort during catheter insertion and bladder filling.

Equipment

- A 14 French straight urinary catheter
- Sterile urinary catheterization tray
- 50-ml catheter-tip syringe without the piston
- 1 liter of sterile water
- A fracture pan or urinal

- A measuring hat or cap for the toilet bowl
- A nearby toilet or bedside commode
- Small absorbent peri pads
- Food coloring for easier detection of urinary incontinence (optional).

Procedure

1. Begin by observing the patient void into the measuring hat set in the toilet. Note any voiding difficulties (e.g., hesitancy, straining—and the voided volume). Straining may indicate that the patient has a detrusor weakness that can predispose the patient to postoperative urinary retention.
2. Note the effect that straining has on the force of the urinary stream and the patient's ability to interrupt the voiding midstream. The former (force of stream) will decrease during straining for patients with detrusor sphincter dysynergia (DSD). The latter evaluates the patient for potential success with pelvic muscle exercises.
3. Position the patient on a fracture pan or have the urinal nearby to measure any leakage during the filling.
4. Within 5 to 10 minutes of the patient's voiding, catheterize the patient for a postvoid residual. Note the ease of insertion and the postvoid residual amount. Residuals greater than 100 cc indicate an underactive detrusor or outflow obstruction. They may also indicate destrusor hyperactivity (DH) with impaired contractility, stress incontinence, or a puddling of urine in a cystocele.
5. Attach the 50-ml syringe tip to the free end of the urinary catheter and hold it upright at approximately 15 cm above the pubic symphysis.
6. Begin filling the syringe in 50-ml increments with the sterile water.
7. Record the volume instilled when the patient feels the first urge to void and then when maximum bladder capacity is achieved. The latter is the point at which the patient feels unable to hold any more or when an involuntary nonstrained bladder contrac-

tion occurs, noted by a persistent upward movement greater than or equal to 15 cm of water pressure in the syringe or leakage around the catheter. Normally the first urge occurs after 150 to 350 ml of water is instilled and the normal bladder capacity is 300 to 600 ml.

8. Note whether the patient can inhibit the contraction and note the amount of incontinence.
9. Remove the catheter and bedpan and ask the patient to hold the fluid in the bladder.
10. With the bladder now full, place a peri pad over the urethra. Have the patient cough forcefully 3 to 5 times while sitting and 3 to 5 times while standing and observe for any incontinence. If incontinence occurs note the amount and timing in relation to the cough (i.e., during or shortly after). Urinary leakage with coughing suggests stress incontinence, whereas urinary leakage that is delayed for more than a few seconds suggests urge incontinence. It is important to have the patient relax and spread the legs during this procedure and not to test for this during an urge to void.
11. Finally, have the patient empty the bladder into the measuring hat. Again, observe for any voiding difficulty and note the amount voided. Subtract this amount from the total amount instilled to get the calculated postvoid residual.

Practitioner Followup/Complications

The most significant risk to the patient is for a urinary tract infection (UTI). For this reason the urinary catheterization is performed using sterile technique. UTI symptoms include: burning and urgency with urination; increased frequency of urination; and cloudy, strong, or foul-smelling urine. If any of these should occur, this should be reported to the primary care provider. Overall, the incidence of urinary tract infections is quite low and can easily be treated subsequently with oral antibiotics should it occur. To help prevent a UTI from occurring after the procedure, patients should be sure to drink 2 to 3 liters of fluid a day unless they have a medical condition that contraindicates this.

Patients should be referred for further testing when the patient has a known or suspected neurologic disorder in conjunction with the incontinence; has a history of previous corrective surgery for urinary incontinence or radical pelvic surgery or irradiation; or complains of incontinence that cannot be demonstrated clinically, incontinence symptoms that have not resolved with conservative measures within 4 to 6 weeks or improved significantly within 3 to 4 weeks. Patients also should be referred if there is rapid recurrence of a symptomatic urinary tract infection (e.g., fever, suprapubic or flank pain); there is a severe cystocele or rectocele; there is marked prostatic enlargement or suspicion of cancer; there is severe hesitancy, straining, or interrupted urinary stream; the postvoid residual is greater than 100 cc; there is associated perineal or suprapubic pain, hematuria, or difficulty passing the urinary catheter; if the patient is unaware of the urinary incontinence despite a normal mental status, or if the diagnosis remains uncertain.

CPT BILLING CODE
51725–Simple cystometrogram (CMG) (e.g., spinal manometer).

BIBLIOGRAPHY

Brocklehurst JC: Urinary incontinence in old age: helping the general practitioner to make a diagnosis, *Gerontology* 36(Suppl 2):3, 1990.

Brubaker L, Sand PK: Cystometry, urethrocystometry, and video cystourethrography, *Clin Obstet Gynecol* 33(2):315, 1990.

Chancellor MB, Blaivas JG: Diagnostic evaluation of incontinence in patients with neurological disorders, *Comprehensive Ther* 17(2):37, 1991.

Cutner LA, Cardoza L: Urinary incontinence—diagnosis, *Practitioner* 235(1498):24, 1991.

Diokno AC, Weels TJ, Brink CA: Urinary incontinence in elderly women: urodynamic evaluation, *J Am Geriatr Soc* 35(10):940, 1987.

Dubeau CE, Resnick M: Evaluation of the causes and severity of geriatric incontinence, *Urol Clin North Am* 18(2):243, 1991.

Fonda D, Brimage PJ, D'Astoli M: Simple screening for urinary incontinence in the elderly: comparison of simple and multichannel cystometry, *Urology* 42(5):536, 1993.

Ivey JF: Understanding and evaluating chronic urinary incontinence, *J Florida Med Assoc* 79(12): 823, 1992.

Juma S, Little NA, Raz S: Basic evaluation of female urinary incontinence, *Am J Kidney Dis* 16(4):317, 1990.

Ouslander JG, Leach GE, Staskin DR: Simplified tests of lower urinary tract function in the evaluation of geriatric urinary incontinence, *J Am Geriatri Soc* 37(8):706, 1989.

Resnick NM: Noninvasive diagnosis of the patient with complex incontinence, *Gerontology* 36(Suppl 2):8, 1990.

Sand PK, Bubaker LT, Novak, T: Simple standing incremental cystometry as a screening method for detrusor instability, *Obstet Gynecol* 77(3):453, 1991.

CHAPTER 9

Gynecologic Procedures

Papanicolaou Smear Test

Description

This procedure obtains smears of the cervix and the vagina (although smears from the vulva and endometrium may also be obtained) for cytologic examination. The test is used principally for the diagnosis of precancerous and cancerous conditions, for hormonal assessment, and for the diagnosis of inflammatory diseases. This test may be performed at any time that heavy menstrual bleeding is not present but is best done in midcycle in a woman who has not had intercourse for 24 hours and has not placed any substances in her vagina for at least 48 hours.

Indications

Pap smears are indicated annually for all women by age 18 or after onset of sexual activity.

Pap smears should be done for all women on their initial visit for prenatal care and at 6 weeks postpartum.

High-risk women may require earlier and more frequent testing. Risk factors include:

- Early onset of sexual activity (under age 18)
- Multiple sexual partners

- Tobacco smoking
- History of illicit drug use (IV or oral)
- History of genital condylomata
- History of other sexually transmitted diseases
- Sexual partner with genital condylomata
- Sexual partner with more than three sexual partners (lifetime)
- History of abnormal Pap smear
- Diethyl stilbesterol (DES) exposed in utero

Contraindications/Precautions

There are no absolute contraindications to Pap smears.

Relative contraindications usually involve situations that make obtaining or interpreting a Pap difficult. These include:

- Medications such as tetracycline and digitalis
- Use of lubricating jelly
- Douching, intercourse, or vaginal medications within 24 hours of a Pap smear collection
- Active vaginitis or cervicitis
- Pelvic inflammatory disease
- Menstrual flow

These conditions may yield a higher percentage of unsatisfactory specimens, often making repeat studies necessary. If possible, defer a Pap to a more favorable time. If not, to reduce patient anxiety, advise her of the possibility that this test may have to be repeated.

Patient Preparation/Education

Practitioners explain the purpose and procedure of exam, and answer any questions the patient may have.

Practitioners should tell the patient that she may experience slight discomfort when the cervix is manipulated and the specimen is collected.

Just before the test, the practitioner should ask the patient to empty her bladder.

The patient should remove all clothing (except socks and shoes).

Appropriate drapes should be provided.

Equipment

- Exam table suitable for placing patient in lithotomy position
- Well-lighted, warm room with additional "focused" light source
- Cloth or paper drapes
- Two pair of nonsterile gloves
- Various sized speculums
- Method for warming speculum if using metal
- Cytobrush
- Cotton tipped applicators
- Wood spatula
- Glass slide (frosted on one end)
- Appropriate patient identification and history forms
- Lead pencil
- Fixative
- Culture or transport media and swabs for collection of *Gonorrhea, Chlamydia,* Herpes, fungal and KOH/wet mount specimens
- Ring forceps, cervical tenaculum, or cervical hook (rarely needed)

Procedure

1. Obtain the patient's history, review the systems, and answer her questions. Clarify her risk factors for cervical dysplasia.
2. Proceed with the rest of the exam (breast and general physical exams), leaving the pelvic examination for last.
3. Label the frosted end of the glass slide with the patient's name and other identifying data; ensure that all appropriate paperwork is complete and that other culture specimen tubes are present and labeled as needed.
4. Adjust the lighting.
5. Assist her into the lithotomy position.
6. Wearing gloves, begin the examination. Inspect the vulva, assessing hair pattern, anatomy, estrogen effect, discharge, and Bartholins and Skeins glands.
7. Lubricate the speculum with warm water and insert it into the vagina with a gentle posterior pressure, exposing the cervix. Adjust the speculum to obtain adequate visualization of the cervix and tighten the screw or lock the speculum open.

Encourage the patient to relax and breath through her mouth. Inspect the cervix, looking for inflammation or infection. Avoid rubbing or otherwise traumatizing the cervix.

8. Identify cervical landmarks, including the transformation zone and the squamocolumnar junction. Note the nature of the cervical mucus, gently blotting excess mucus or discharge. Examine for any gross lesions (i.e., erosions, leukoplakia, Nabothian cysts, condylomata).

9. First obtain an endocervical scraping by rotating a cytobrush 180 degrees in the endocervical canal. Then gently rotate a wooden spatula in a circular fashion over the entire transformation zone. Sampling the vaginal pool is of little benefit unless the patient has had a hysterectomy. In this case, be sure to sample the vaginal cuff as well.

10. Smear the wooden spatula sample on the glass slide first and then quickly apply the Cytobrush sample. Spray a fixative or place the slide in a glass container with ethyl alcohol (ETOH) immediately (within 5 seconds).

11. Obtain appropriate cervical cultures after cytologic sampling has been completed.

12. Slowly withdraw the speculum, examining the vaginal walls as the speculum is removed. Note any abnormalities.

13. Complete the remainder of the bimanual exam.

14. Change gloves and perform a rectal exam on all women over age 40.

15. Once the specimens are obtained, assist the patient as needed to redress.

Interpretation of results

Adequacy: The Pap report should indicate whether the smear has been adequate. Ordinarily, the reporting of endocervical cells along with squamous cells implies adequate sampling. The term "squamous metaplasia" has the same significance as reporting "endocervical cells present." Either report indicates that the transformation zone has been sampled. This therefore implies that an adequate sample has been taken.

Interpretation system: Using the Bethesda system, interpretations are as follows:

Normal: No abnormal cells are present.

Atypia: Atypical cells are present, but no neoplasia.

Low-grade squamous intraepithelial lesion (SIL) [HPV changes and cervical intraepithelial neoplasia (CIN) I]: Smear contains abnormal cells consistent with dysplasia.

High-grade SIL [CIN II, CIN III, carcinoma in situ (CIS)]: Smear contains abnormal cells consistent with carcinoma in situ.

Invasive carcinoma: Smear contains abnormal cells consistent with carcinoma of squamous origin.

Indications for colposcopy

Indications for colposcopy are:

1. Pap report findings of:

   - Persistent squamous atypia.
   - Dysplasia of any degree (CIN I through III, low- or high-grade SIL)
   - Evidence of malignant cells
   - Evidence of HPV infection
   - Evidence of glandular atypia

2. Pelvic exam findings of:

   - Abnormal-appearing cervix
   - Abnormal-feeling cervix
   - Genital condylomata at any site.

3. Other indications:

   - Positive HPV-DNA screen
   - DES offspring
   - Partner with genital condylomata
   - History of sexual abuse
   - History of sexually transmitted disease.

Postprocedure patient education

Notify the patient that some women experience some light pink, painless spotting for 24 hours after the procedure.

Inform the patient about the methods used in your facility to followup test results (Pap smear, cultures, etc.).

Recommend that the patient have Pap tests done at least annually, and that sometimes more frequent testing is necessary.

Practitioner Followup/Complications

Practitioners should be knowledgeable regarding the results of the exam in order to completely answer any questions the patient may have. It should for remembered that a suspicious test does not mean that the patient has cancer.

CPT BILLING CODES
99070—Pap smear.
88150—Pap smear interpretation.

BIBLIOGRAPHY

Beal MW: Understanding cervical cytology, *Nurse Practitioner* 12(3):8, 1987.
Benson RC, Pernoll ML: *Handbook of obstetrics & gynecology*, ed 9, New York, 1994, McGraw-Hill.
Boon ME, de Graff Guilloud JC, Rietveld WJ: Analysis of five sampling methods for the preparation of cervical smears, *Int Acad Cytol* 1(6):843, 1989.
Boon ME and others: Exploiting the "toothpick effect" of the cytobrush by plastic embedding of cervical samples, *Int Acad Cytol* 35(1):57, 1990.
Hatcher RA and others: *Contraceptive technology*, 16th rev ed, New York, 1993, Irvington.
Hoffman MS, Gordy LW, Cavanagh D: Use of the cytobrush for cervical sampling after cryotherapy, *Int Acad Cytol* 79, 1990.
Macgregor JE: What constitutes an adequate cervical smear? *Br J Obstet Gynecol* 98:6, 1991.
Pairwuti S: False-negative papanicolaou smears for women with cancerous and precancerous lesions of the uterine cervix, *Int Acad Cytol* 35(1):40, 1991.
Rammou-Kinia R, Anagnostopoulou I, Gomousa M: Comparison of spatual and non-spatual methods for cervical sampling, *Int Acad Cytol,* 35(1):69, 1989.
The revised Bethesda system for reporting cervical/vaginal cytologic diagnosis: report of the 1991 Bethesda workshop, *J Reprod Med* 37(5):282, 1992.

The Wet Mount

Description

The wet mount, a simple microscopic procedure, is the most useful technique available for the diagnosis of certain vaginal infections. It should be performed on all patients with vaginal symptoms, even if the diagnosis seems obvious. This is an accessory tool to the history, the inspection of the vulvar and vaginal mucosa, and the determination of the pH of the vaginal secretions.

Indications

Indications for making a wet mount are:

- Vaginal discharge
- Vulvar or vaginal pruritus
- Vulvar or vaginal pain
- Malodorous vaginal secretions

Contraindications/Precautions

There are no absolute contraindications to wet mounts. Relative contraindications include recent douching, intravaginal medications, or menses.

Patient Preparation/Education

Practitioners explain the purpose and procedure of the exam and answer any questions.

Just before the test, the practitioner asks the patient to empty her bladder.

The practitioner asks the patient to remove her clothing from the waist down.

The practitioner assists the patient into the lithotomy position and drapes her with a sheet.

Equipment

- Exam table suitable for placing patient in the lithotomy position
- Well-lit, warm room with additional "focused" light source
- Cloth or paper drapes
- Two pairs of nonsterile gloves
- Variously sized specula

- Method for warming speculum, if using a metal one
- Cotton-tipped applicators
- Glass slides and coverslips
- Small test tubes
- Culture media or tubes for collecting *Chlamydia* and *Gonorrhea* specimens
- Normal saline solution
- 10% KOH solution
- Microscope
- pH test tape
- Appropriate patient identification and history forms

Procedure

1. Gently insert the vaginal speculum (no lubricants, except water, should be used) and visualize the vaginal walls and cervix, noting any lesions, erosions, ulcerations, leukoplakia, or condylomata. Observe the vaginal discharge—note the amount, the color, and any odor.
2. Collect a copious amount of vaginal discharge with a cotton swab and place it in a tube containing 1 ml of normal saline. Vigorously mix the swab in the saline.
3. The pH test tape may be used to screen for specific types of vaginitis. A piece of the test tape may be directly applied to the vaginal wall, or the tape can be touched to the speculum after it's removed. The following conditions are indicated at the pH:

   Normal flora: pH under 4
   Candidiasis: pH 4 to 5
   Bacterial vaginosis: pH 5 to 6
   Trichomonas pH 6 to 7

4. Obtain Specimens from the cervix for culture of *Chlamydia* and *Gonorrhea* at the same time that wet smear specimens are obtained. Insert the appropriate applicators directly into the cervical canal until the tip is completely inside the os. Gently twirl the tip several times in the os (leaving it in there for several seconds to absorb organisms). Withdraw the applicator and place in the proper containers.

5. Remove the speculum and do a bimanual exam if it is indicated.
6. Place one large drop of saline mixture in the centers of two glass slides (or on each end of one slide, if preferred).
7. Add 1 drop of KOH to one specimen and sniff it immediately for the characteristic "fishy" odor of bacterial vaginosis.
8. Cover both specimens with coverslips. Plan to view the plain saline specimen first, to allow time for the KOH to lyse cells before looking for *Candida*.
9. With the 10× lens in place, using low-power light, and with the condenser in the lowest position, place the slide on the stage and lower the objective until it is as close to the slide as possible.
10. Adjust the eyepieces until a single round field is seen. Turn the coarse-focus knob until the specimen is focused. Use the fine-focus knob to bring the specimen into sharp focus.
11. Examine the slide in a systematic manner, until you have a general impression of the number of squamous cells.
12. Switch to high power (40×); it may be necessary to increase the amount of light slightly.
13. Evaluate the slide for vaginal epithelial cells (flat with sharp, clear edges), clue cells (epithelial cells covered with bacteria obscuring the edges of the cell and giving the cell a granular appearance), bacteria (normal vaginal bacteria), lactobacilli, (large rods), WBCs (a few are normal but should not exceed the number of epithelial cells), *Trichomonas* (ovoid, flagellated organisms recognizable by their motility) and *Candida* (branching pseudohyphae). Even if one organism is identified, continue to scan the slide systematically to evaluate the specimen fully. Vaginitis may have multiple causes.
14. Move to the KOH slide. Switch back to low power to scan the slide for *Candida*. If hyphae are noted, switch to high power to confirm the impression.
15. Be sure to wipe any spilled fluid from the stage. If the objective becomes contaminated, use only special lens paper to clean it.

Interpretation of results

Table 9-1 displays interpretation of results for wet mounts.

Table 9-1

Wet Mount Interpretations

	Physiological	Candida	Gardnerella	Trichomonas	Atrophia
Symptoms	None	Pruritus, burning	May have pruritus, burning	May have pruritus	Vulvar, vaginal dryness
Malodor	None	Yeast smell	Fishy or musty	Variable	Variable
Increased mucosal erythema	None	Yes	May or may not have this	Yes	May or may not have this
Consistency	Floccular	Thick, curdlike	Thin, creamy	Copious, frothy	Mucoid, blood tinged
pH	3.5–4.1	3.5–4.5	5–6	6–7	As high as 7.0
Wet smear	Rare WBCs, large gm+ rods; squamous epithelial cells	Budding filaments spores, pseudohyphae	Clue cells	Copious WBCs, trichomonads	Copious WBCs, parabasal, and intermediate cells; paucity of superficial cells
KOH	None	Budding filaments, spores, pseudohyphae	Fishy odor, musty odor		
Treatment of choice	None	Imidazole derivative	Metronidazole	Metronidazole	Estrogen cream

Gm+, gram positive.

Postprocedure patient education

Provide the patient with medication instructions if they are needed, including side effects and the importance of completing the medication as directed.

Discuss the need for followup appointments with the patient.

Discuss the need for partner treatment if necessary.

Discuss the appropriate timing for the resumption of sexual activity.

Practitioner Followup/Complications

Practitioners should call the patient with any positive culture reports.

Practitioners should be prepared to offer alternative medications if medication side effects are extreme.

CPT BILLING CODES

58999—Wet smear and KOH preparation.

BIBLIOGRAPHY

Gant NF, Cunningham FG: *Basic gynecology and obstetrics,* Norwalk, Conn, 1993, Appleton & Lange.

Lichtman R, Papera S: *Gynecology: well woman care,* Norwalk, Conn, 1990, Appleton & Lange.

Treatment of Condylomata Acuminata

Description

Condylomata acuminata (venereal warts) is a sexually transmitted disease that has become alarmingly prevalent in recent years. Because of the close association with cervical cancer, venereal warts are of increasing concern to health care providers. Genital HPV (human papilloma virus) is caused by virus types 6, 11, 16, 18, 31, 33, and 35. The HPV types that are considered "high risk" for malignant potential include all types above 16 because they are more often associated in high-grade lesions and in cervical squamous and adenocarcinomas. All are characterized by the formation of warty growths primarily in the anongenital region. The incubation period is 1 to 6 months but may be much longer (up to 30 years). The usual incubation period is 3 weeks to 3 months after exposure.

The typical presentation of condylomata acuminata is 2 to 3 mm in diameter and 10 to 15 mm in height, soft, sessile or papillary swellings that may occur singly or in clusters. Infection of long duration may create cauliflower-like mass.

Warts are usually flesh colored or slightly darker in caucasians, black in dark-skinned patients, and brownish in Asians. Lymphadenopathy is usually absent.

On moist skin areas, such as the vagina or vaginal introitus, warts may have the appearance of multiple, fine, fingerlike projections. On the cervix, they appear as flat-topped papules 1 to 4 mm in size.

On nonmucosal dry areas, the warts appear as squared-off keratotic papules.

Giant condylomata acuminata appear as round, large, soft papules or nodules with a pebbly strawberry appearance.

HPV may invade both external and internal surfaces, so particular caution needs to be taken to examine the entire lower genital tract for lesions. These lesions may or may not be visible to the naked eye, so if there is any suspicion of condylomata infection, colposcopy of the genital area after application of acetic acid is very valuable in diagnosis.

Condylomata tend to increase in both number and size during pregnancy and in association with immunodeficiency or poor hygiene, but the natural history is unpredictable. Left untreated, they may regress spontaneously or persist and spread. All methods of treating HPV have significant failure and recurrence rates.

Indications

Indications for treatment are:

- Visible, acuminata condylomata
- Symptomatic condylomata

Contraindications/Precautions

Practitioners do not treat if there is any known adverse reaction to the selected treatment modality.

Practitioners do not treat any lesion that may be cancerous (These lesions should be biopsied before ablation).

For treatment options, see Table 9-2.

Because many of these remain surgical procedures, primary care practitioners commonly limit their treatment to the chemical ablation methods described below.

Patient Preparation/Education

Practitioners explain the procedure to the patient, being sure to discuss its risks and benefits, and answer any questions.

The practitioner assists the female client into the dorsal lithotomy position and drapes her appropriately; a mirror can be offered to the patient so that she may learn how to inspect and identify warts

Practitioners should explain that the application of chemicals will cause a sharp stinging pain that will last about 5 minutes.

Equipment

- 3% to 5% acetic acid (full-strength white vinegar) for identifying lesions
- Several large "scopette" swabs
- 85% trichloroacetic acid (TCA) or 0.5% Podofilox for treating lesions
- Several cotton-tipped applicators

Procedure

1. Using a large scopette swab dipped in acetic acid, generously swab the external genitalia. Leave on for 3 to 5 minutes. Acetowhitening or blanching of lesions will occur. This is very important in identifying all areas to treat.

Table 9-2

Treatments for Condylomata Acuminata

Therapy	Clearance rates (%)	Recurrence rates (%)	Pain	Number of visits	Anesthesia	Use in pregnancy	Cost
Podophyllin	22–77	11–74	Mild to moderate	3	No	No	$ 183
Podofilox	45–50	21–33	Mild		No	No	
Trichloroacetic acid (TCA)	81	36	Moderate	3	No	Yes	$ 183
Cryotherapy	63–88	21–40	Moderate	3	No	Yes	$ 285
Surgery	93	29	Moderate	2	Yes	Yes	$ 340
Electrodesiccation	94	22	Moderate	2	Yes	Yes	$ 340
Interferon	19–62	21–25	Moderate	9–18	No	No	$1500
Laser	31–94	3–95	Moderate	1	Yes	Yes	$2650

2. While the acetic acid is working on external lesions, gently insert the speculum and inspect the vaginal and cervical surfaces. If there is no history of a recent Pap smear, obtain a Pap and any indicated vaginal or cervical cultures. Paint the vagina and cervix with acetic acid and look for white patches representing HPV.

3. Using a regular cotton-tipped wooden stick applicator, apply TCA directly onto the visible wart surface. Avoid getting the solution on normal skin. For smaller lesions, use the wooden end to apply treatment, and for larger lesions use the cotton-tipped end. Treated warts develop a white appearance several seconds after the application of TCA. Avoid contact of healthy skin against the treated surface. The treated areas should slough in 1 to 2 days. Patients may need retreatment every 2 weeks until the lesions disappear.

4. Teach the patient how to apply topical Podofilox solution at home to treat external genital warts. Podofilox is a pure compound and does not contain the toxic substances that podophyllin does, but it is not to be used on mucous membrane or perianal tissue. The patient should apply Podofilox with cotton-tipped applicators soaked with the medication twice a day for three consecutive days, using no more than 0.5 cc each day. Then the patient must wait 4 days before starting the cycle again. This process may continue for a maximum of 6 weeks or until no warts are visible. The entire process can be repeated at a later time if more warts appear.

Postprocedure patient education

Instruct the patient to watch for and report any signs of infection.

Treated areas should be washed and dried gently each day of the healing process.

Advise the patient to return to the clinic for evaluation and additional application of TCA, if necessary, in 7 to 10 days.

Advise patient to refer her sexual partners for exam and treatment (85% of exposed partners have or will develop genital warts).

Recurrence is possible without reinfection, because treatment does not always eradicate very small warts.

Advise the patient to use condoms during therapy or until complete colinical cure is obtained.

If the patient is starting a new relationship, discuss both partner's sexual and medical histories.

Stress the importance of an annual gynecologic examination with Pap smear.

Practitioner Followup/Complications

If the area treated at one visit is too large, extensive necrosis and pain may occur. Reasonably sized areas should be treated over multiple visits.

Recurrence or persistence of the lesions is common.

CPT BILLING CODES

17100—Destruction by any method, including laser, of benign skin lesions other than cutaneous vascular proliferative lesions on any area other than the face; including local anesthesia; one lesion.

17101—Destruction by any method, including laser, of benign skin lesions other than cutaneous vascular proliferative lesions on any area other than the face; including local anesthesia; second lesion.

17102—Destruction by any method, including laser, of benign skin lesions other than cutaneous vascular proliferative lesions on any area other than the face; including local anesthesia; over two lesions, each additional lesion up to 15 lesions.

17104—Destruction by any method, including laser, of benign skin lesions other than cutaneous vascular proliferative lesions on any area other than the face; including local anesthesia; 15 or more lesions.

17105—Destruction by any method, including laser, of benign skin lesions other than cutaneous vascular proliferative lesions on any area other than the face; including local anesthesia; complicated or extensive lesions.

46900—Destruction of lesion(s); anus (e.g., condyloma), simple; chemical.

46924—Destruction of lesion(s); anus, extensive; any method.

56501—Destruction of lesion(s); vulva, simple; any method.

56515—Destruction of lesion(s); extensive, any method.

57061—Destruction of vaginal lesion(s); simple; any method.

57065—Destruction of vaginal lesion(s); extensive, any method.

BIBLIOGRAPHY

Friedman-Kien A, Oi R, Reid R: Genital warts: nusiance or menace? *Patient Care* August 15, 1988, p. 36.

Hatcher RA and others: *Contraceptive technology;* rev ed 16, New York, 1994, Irvington.

Hawkins J, Roberto J, Haney J: *Protocols for nurse practitioners in gynecologic settings,* ed 3, New York, 1991, The Tiresias Press.

Nettina S, Kauffman F: Diagnosis and management of sexually transmitted genital lesions, *Nurse Practitioner* 15(1):20, 1990.

Rapini R: Venereal warts, *Primary Care* 17(1):127, 1990.

Pessary Use

Description

Vaginal pessaries are an ancient medical therapy and can be considered a "modern" type of diaphragm. Today, they are made of rubber or plastic and often include a metal band or spring-type frame. Many different forms of pessaries have been developed over the years, but fewer than a dozen have unique properties or are specifically helpful. Pessaries are used primarily to support the uterus, the cervical stump, or hernias of the pelvic floor and are effective because they increase the tension of the pelvic floor. Some types of medicated vaginal suppositories act as pessaries as well.

Indications

GYNECOLOGIC

Pessaries are used for genital hernias or uterine prolapse in high-risk patients or patients who refuse surgery.

Pessaries assist in healing cervical decubitus ulcers associated with uterine prolapse before corrective surgery.

A pessary may help reduce cystocele or rectocele.

A pessary may alleviate menorrhagia, dysmenorrhea, or dyspareunia caused by uterine retroposition or adnexal prolapse.

A pessary might also be used as a test to see whether hysteropexy will relieve backache caused by retroversion.

Pessaries have been used with increasing frequency to control urinary stress incontinence by exerting pressure beneath the urethra or by improving the posterior ureterovesical angle.

In infertility management, a pessary may be used to tilt the cervix into a more midplane position (especially in anterior position cervixes).

Surgeons may use pessaries to assist in surgery by holding the uterus in one position.

OBSTETRICAL

Pessaries may be used to prevent threatened abortion thought to be caused by marked uterine retroversion.

Pessaries may be used to promote healing of cervical ulcers caused by prolapse in pregnancy.

They may be helpful in relieving acute urinary retention caused by retroversion in midpregnancy.

Relief or prevention of postpartum subinvolution or retroversion may also be achieved by pessaries.

Some providers use pessaries to protect against spontaneous abortion in cervical incompetence.

Contraindications/Precautions

Pessaries are contraindicated in acute genital tract infections and in adherent retroversion of the uterus.

Patient Preparation/Education

Practitioners discuss in detail with the patient the reasons a pessary is being considered and how it will benefit this individual patient. Practitioners should be careful to inform the patient that pessaries do NOT cure uterine prolapse, but that they may be used for months or years for relief of symptoms under proper supervision.

Practitioners explain the fitting procedure and proper pessary use and answer any questions.

Equipment

- Lubricant
- Nonsterile gloves
- Exam table

Table 9-3 describes various pessary devices.

Procedure

1. Before fitting the pessary, perform a Pap smear and pelvic exam to rule out cervical or vaginal infections.
2. Explain the procedure to the patient; have her get into the lithotomy position. Offer her a mirror so that she may watch the fitting process and explain the insertion process step by step as you go through the pessary fitting.
3. Perform a bimanual exam noting length, shape, and position of the cervix, vagina, and uterus.
4. Choose a pessary designed to alleviate the symptoms this particular woman is having (see Table 9-3 and Figs. 9-1 and 9-2).
5. Correct fit is somewhat subjective but very important: Too large a pessary can cause irritation and ulceration, and one that is too small may not stay in place or may protrude. There should be

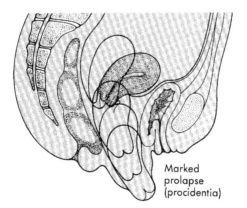

Marked prolapse (procidentia)

Fig. 9-1 Depiction of prolapse of uterus. (From Beare PG, Myers J: *Principles and practice of adult health nursing,* ed 2, St Louis, 1994, Mosby.

Table 9-3

Pessary Devices

Types	Description
Hodge	Elongated, curved ovoid; one end is placed behind the symphysis and the other in the posterior vaginal fornix. The anterior bow is curved, avoiding the urethra, the cervix rests in the larger posterior bow. This type of pessary is used to hold the uterus in place after it has been surgically repositioned.
Gellhorn and Mange	Shaped like a button; provides a ringlike surface for the cervix to rest on. It also has a "stem" that rests on the perineal floor to stabilize it. These types correct a significant uterine prolapse and are used if there is still some reasonable perineal support.
Gehrung	This pessary resembles two elongated letter Cs with crossbars between them. The cervix is supported between the long arms and the device arches the anterior vaginal wall. This is helpful in reducing cystoceles.
Ring	Can be made of "rigid" or soft "doughnut" material. This stretches the vagina and elevates the cervix. This type of pessary is helpful in reducing both cystocele and rectocele.
Ball or bee cell	Hollow plastic "ball" or sponge rubber "bee cell" ball acts like the ring pessary in supporting the cystocele and rectocele. Moderate perineal support is required to keep these pessaries in place.
Napier	Cup and stem network supported by an external "belt" system. Elevates the cervix and uterus. Used for marked prolapse and in cases where surgery is necessary but the patient may not tolerate the operation.
Inflatable	Much like a ring pessary; the ball, however, is inflatable. When the valve inside the stem is in the "down" position, air inflates the device; when the valve is "up" the air is sealed in and inflation is stable. Assists in reducing cystocele and rectocele.

room for one finger width on all sides of the pessary frame and the vaginal wall, but no part of the pessary should be visible at the introitus.

6. Instruct the woman on pessary insertion and removal, allowing plenty of time for practice. She should be asked to stand, walk, and squat to determine; (1) whether pain occurs, (2) whether the

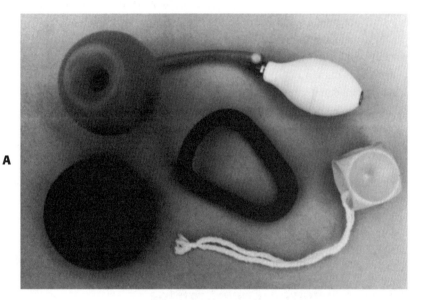

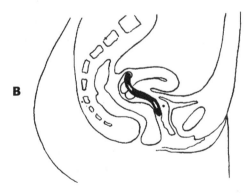

Fig. 9-2 A Examples of pessaries (Smith-Hodge, donut, inflatable types). **B** Pessary in place to hold posterior vaginal fornix and, with it, attached cervix wall backward and upward in pelvis. (A from Droegemuller W and others: *Comprehensive gynecology,* St Louis, 1987, Mosby. B from Beacham DW, Beacham WD: *Synopsis of gynecology,* ed 10, St Louis, 1982, Mosby.)

pessary becomes displaced, or (3) whether the uterus remains in the desired position.

Postprocedure patient education

Vaginal odor or discharge can occur and may be decreased by soaking the device in 1 teaspoon of apple cider vinegar mixed in 1 quart of water, by performing low-pressure acetic acid douches, or by use of acidic vaginal creams.

All pessaries should be removed and cleaned at least monthly, and some forms need to be removed nightly (bee cell and inflatable) for cleaning and to protect vaginal mucosa from the effects of constant pressure.

Instruct the patient to wash the pessary with warm soap and water and not to use any talc or perfumed powders.

If vaginal infection occurs, the patient should soak the pessary in rubbing alcohol for 20 minutes before reuse.

Advise the patient to bring the device with her to her annual gynecologic exam to evaluate its fit.

Pessaries should be reevaluated for appropriate fit after pregnancy, miscarriage, or abortion.

Practitioner Followup/Complications

Practitioners should be available to answer any questions, especially in the first 2 to 3 months of initial pessary use.

Practitioners schedule a 2 week followup exam to check fit and placement.

Practitioners and patients should consider annual pessary replacements to avoid problems with rubber or plastic deterioration.

Toxic shock is a theoretical, but unreported complication.

Vaginal lacerations or abrasions can occur if the pessary is improperly fitted or left in place without periodic cleaning.

CPT BILLING CODE
57160—Insertion of pessary.

BIBLIOGRAPHY

Gant NF, Cunningham FG: *Basic gynecology and obstetrics,* Norwalk, Conn, 1993, Appleton & Lange.

Hacker NF, Moore JG: *Essentials of obstetrics and gynecology,* ed 2, Philadelphia, 1992, WB Saunders.

Stewart F and others: *Understanding your body—every woman's guide to gynecology and health,* New York, 1987, Bantam.

Diaphragm Fitting

Description

The diaphragm is one type of barrier contraceptive method. Barrier contraceptives are possibly the oldest contraceptive devices, with natural sea sponges probably being the most ancient. The diaphragm was introduced in the United States in the early 1900s and rapidly became "the" modern contraceptive device. It has essentially remained unchanged since then; only the addition of spermicide and the development of a "wide-seal" style have altered it at all.

Diaphragms work by mechanically blocking sperm from entering the cervix. When used with a spermicidal jelly, the theoretical contraceptive effectiveness approaches 98%, although in actual use the effectiveness drops to 80% to 93% for new users and to 97% for long-term users.

Indications

Diaphragms are indicated when there is a desire for rapidly reversible contraception without hormonal influences.

Diaphragms are indicated for inability or unwillingness to use other contraceptive methods.

Diaphragms aid in sexually transmitted disease (STD) protection in addition to hormonal contraceptive use.

Contraindications/Precautions

Diaphragms should not be used in patients who lack motivation.

Diaphragms cannot be used when there are abnormalities in vaginal or pelvic anatomy that interfere with fit or stable placement.

Latex allergy contraindicates diaphragm use.

Inability to learn the proper insertion technique also contraindicates use.

A history of toxic shock syndrome is a contraindication.

A patient who is uncomfortable touching her own vagina will not use the diaphragm.

Fitting sooner than 6 weeks postpartum or before completed involution is to be avoided.

A large cystocele or rectocele contraindicates diaphragm use.

Uterine prolapse also contraindicates use.

Diaphragms should not be used when there is repeated urinary tract infection that persists despite attempts to refit the diaphragm. A patient with a history of recurrent UTIs may opt to choose another method.

Patient Preparation/Education

Practitioners discuss in detail all available contraceptive choices with the patient, discussing the advantages and disadvantages of each.

Practitioners explain the fitting procedure and proper diaphragm use, including contraceptive effectiveness statistics, and answer any questions.

Equipment

- Diaphragm fitting kit (contains diaphragms varying in size from 55 to 95 mm circumference, in 5 mm increments).
- Diaphragm types:

  Arching spring: Forms an arc when compressed. Good for women with relaxed pelvic support, cystocele, or rectocele. The firmer rim makes insertion easier. This is the most popular diaphragm in the United States.

  Coil spring: Firm spring strength; best for women with average vaginal tone and with average pubic arch depth.

  Flat spring: Gentle spring strength; comfortable for women with very firm vaginal tone. Recommended for smaller women with narrow or shallow pubic arches. Excellent choice for nulliparous women.

- Lubricant
- Exam gloves
- Lithotomy table

Procedure

Before fitting the diaphragm, determine when the last Pap smear was done. If indicated, repeat the Pap and pelvic exam to rule out cervical or vaginal infections.

Explain the procedure to the patient; have her get into the lithotomy position. Offer her a mirror so that she may watch the fitting process and explain the insertion process step by step as you go through the diaphragm fitting.

To determine an approximate diaphragm size:

1. Insert your index and middle fingers into the patient's vagina until your middle finger reaches the posterior wall of the vagina.
2. Use the tip of your thumb to mark the point at which your index finger touches the pubic bone.

   The diaphragm is sized correctly if its opposite rim lies in front of your thumb when you place the diaphragm rim on the tip of your middle finger. (Some providers use an empirical approach and begin with a 75-mm diaphragm because most women wear a 70 to 80 mm diaphragm.)
3. Insert a sample diaphragm in the chosen size by bending the diaphragm in half and sliding it down the posterior wall of the vagina. Aim the entering part of the diaphragm high in the vagina up behind the cervix to lie in the posterior fornix.
4. Check the diaphragm fit by moving your finger around the entire rim of the diaphragm, making sure that it lies in the posterior fornix and snugly behind the pubic bone.
5. The patient should find a properly sized diaphragm comfortable. She should not feel the diaphragm when walking, standing, sitting, or voiding. Have her try each diaphragm in all these positions.
6. It is wise to try a diaphragm one size larger and one size smaller. Choose the largest size diaphragm that is comfortable for the patient and fits snugly in the vagina.

7. To remove the diaphragm hook one finger under the rim of the diaphragm, and it will fold over on itself. Another method is to slide a finger over the rim to break the suction (this is the method women who have longer finger nails will want to use).
8. Have the patient practice and demonstrate insertion and removal. Women may facilitate insertion by placing one leg up on a stool, by squatting, or by laying on their backs with knees bent. The patient should make sure the diaphragm is in the proper position after insertion.

Postprocedure patient education

Teach the patient the anatomy of the vagina. Utilizing a model, assist the patient in learning and identifying landmarks. She should check the position of the diaphragm by inserting her fingers into the vagina. If she cannot reach the posterior fornix, she can feel to make sure that the cervix is covered by the latex dome of the diaphragm and that the anterior rim is under the symphysis pubis.

Instruct her to check the diaphragm for leaks before each use by holding it up to a light or by seeing whether it will hold water.

Instruct the patient to place approximately 1 teaspoon of contraceptive jelly in the dome of the diaphragm and to spread a small amount around the rim. The jelly should come in contact with the cervix.

The diaphragm must stay in place for 6 hours after intercourse. If intercourse is repeated while the diaphragm is in place, additional spermicidal jelly or foam should be inserted into the vagina. It is recommended that the diaphragm not stay in place for more than 24 hours.

Only contraceptive jelly or water-based lubricants should be used. Oil-based products will destroy the latex.

Instruct the patient to wash the diaphragm with mild soap and warm water. It should be stored in the container provided with the diaphragm, in a cool place. Talc and other preparations should not be applied to the diaphragm.

Advise the patient that a diaphragm should be replaced every 2 years, or should be refitted in the event of weight gain or loss of 10 pounds or greater, after the delivery of a child, or in the event of pelvic surgery.

Make the patient aware of the signs and symptoms of toxic shock syndrome: sudden high fever, vomiting, diarrhea, dizziness, faintness, weakness, sore throat, aching muscles and joints, and rash.

Discuss urinary tract infections and diaphragm use. Instruct her to call promptly if she begins to develop urinary tract infection symptoms.

Practitioner Followup/Complications

Practitioners should be prepared to answer telephone questions when prescribing a diaphragm to a new user. Encourage her to call with any problems or concerns.

Pregnancy may occur in new users. If she misses a menstrual cycle, she should obtain a pregnancy test promptly.

CPT BILLING CODE
57170—Diaphragm fitting.

BIBLIOGRAPHY

Hatcher RA, and others: *Contraceptive technology,* ed 16, New York, 1994, Irvington.
Wallace P, producer; Chandler S, director: *fitting the Ortho Diaphragm* (Videotape), The Ortho Pharmaceutical Company, 1989.

Cervical Cap Placement

Description

The cervical cap is another barrier method of contraceptive, which acts similarly to the diaphragm in that it prevents sperm from entering the cervix. A small amount of spermicide is usually placed in the dome to aid in effectiveness, although no studies have been done to document the necessity of this step. It is a small, cup-like, polyurethane device that fits over the cervix and is held in place by suction. Three types of caps are made, but the most popular and widely available in the United States is the cavity rim cap, which is made of rubber and looks much like a thimble (Fig. 9-3).

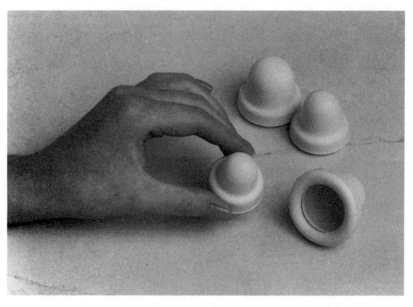

Fig. 9-3 Cervical cap.

This cap is available in four sizes, 22, 25, 28, and 31 mm, with the cap depth increasing as the rim size gets larger. The cervical cap has become increasingly popular in the last decade, largely as a result of women's health organizations.

Indications

Indications for use of a cervical cap are:

- Prevention of pregnancy
- Desire for rapidly reversible contraception without hormonal influences
- Inability or unwillingness to use other contraceptive methods
- STD protection in addition to hormonal contraceptive use

Contraindications/Precautions

Cervical caps should not be used if there is a:

- Lack of motivation
- Patient who is uncomfortable touching her own vagina

- Inability to learn proper insertion technique
- Abnormalities in cervical or vaginal anatomy that interfere with fit or stable placement (e.g., cervical polyps)
- Unresolved or abnormal Pap smear result
- Current vaginal or cervical infection
- Latex allergy
- History of toxic shock syndrome
- Uterine prolapse
- Fitting should not be done sooner than 6 weeks postpartum or before completed involution.

Patient Preparation/Education

Practitioners discuss in detail with the patient all available contraceptive choices, discussing the advantages and disadvantages of each.

Practitioners explain the fitting procedure and proper cervical cap use, including contraceptive effectiveness statistics, and answer any questions.

Equipment

- Cervical cap fitting set that includes one of each of the four sizes of cervical caps (22, 25, 28, and 31 mm)
- Lubricant
- Nonsterile gloves
- Exam table

Procedure

1. Before fitting the cervical cap, perform a Pap smear and pelvic exam to rule out cervical or vaginal infections.
2. Explain the procedure to the patient; have her get into the lithotomy position. Offer her a mirror, so that she may watch the fitting process, and explain the insertion process step by step as you go through the cervical cap fitting.
3. Perform a bimanual exam noting length, shape, and position of

the cervix, as well as any irregularities in the shape of its circumference. Estimate the appropriate cap size.

4. Squeeze the cap rim and insert it, dome outward, into the vagina. Place it over the cervix. Correct fit is somewhat subjective; correct fit can be ascertained if the following criteria are met:

   - The cap covers the entire cervix; no cervix is felt.
   - No space exists between rim and cervix (check ENTIRE circumference to be sure).
   - Suction is adequate and equal on all sides (the cap should not be pulled off easily, and the indentation should remain for at least 30 seconds).
   - Rotation of the cap is not significant; if it does rotate, check to be sure it does not tilt away from the cervix.
   - The dome is midline and faces the introitus (as that penile thrusts will not hit the cap at an angle and dislodge it).
   - The cap is not close to the introitus.

5. Try one size larger and one smaller to confirm the fit of the chosen cap. If two sizes seem appropriate, choose the smaller cap.

6. Instruct the patient on cap insertion and removal, allowing plenty of time for practice. The cap is removed by inserting one or two fingers between the rim and cervix and pulling down and out. Removal is easier if the suction is broken over the posterior rim. When the patient is comfortable with insertion and removal, place the cap on several times, both correctly and incorrectly, and have the patient identify the cap placement and adjust it as necessary.

7. A second visit may be necessary if the patient is having difficulty with insertion or removal. A partner can be taught insertion and removal as well.

Postprocedure patient education

Advise patients to practice insertion and removal before using the cervical cap for contraception the first time. Patients should wear it for 8 hours and check the fit and comfort level.

Instruct patients that, before insertion, they should fill the dome one third full with spermicidal jelly; they should not apply it to the inner rim.

Instruct patients to insert a cervical cap at least ½ hour before intercourse to increase suction.

Advise patients to use a condom along with the cap for the first month of use or first eight acts of intercourse, checking the cap after each use. Patients and their partners should use different sexual positions to see whether the cap will dislodge. If it is dislodged more than once, a smaller size may be necessary or certain sexual positions become unsafe.

Warn patients to allow the cap to remain in place for at least 8 hours after intercourse.

Advise patients not to allow the cap to remain in place longer than 48 hours at a time.

The cap should be washed with warm soap and water. Talc or perfumed powders should not be used.

Patients should check for tears or holes by holding the cap up to the light or filling it with water.

If vaginal infection occurs, the patient should soak the cap in rubbing alcohol for 20 minutes before reuse.

Advise patients to bring the cap to their annual gynecologic exam to evaluate its fit.

Instruct patients not to use cervical caps during menses.

Cervical caps should be refitted after pregnancy, miscarriage, or abortion, and should not be worn in the first 6 weeks postpartum.

Practitioner Followup/Complications

Practitioners should be available to answer any questions, especially in the first 2 to 3 months of initial cap use.

Practitioners schedule a 2 week followup exam to check fit and placement.

The FDA mandates a followup Pap smear 3 months after cap initiation, after which annual Paps are required.

Patients should consider cap replacements annually to avoid problems with cap deterioration.

Toxic shock is a theoretical but unreported complication.

Vaginal lacerations or abrasions can occur if the cap is left in place too long.

Vaginal odor or discharge occurs in 5% to 27% of cap users and may be decreased by soaking the cap in 1 teaspoon apple cider vinegar mixed in 1 quart water or placing a drop of chlorophyll in the dome prior to insertion. Too frequent soaking can deteriorate rubber more rapidly, however.

CPT BILLING CODE

57170—Cervical cap fitting with instructions.

BIBLIOGRAPHY

Hatcher RA, and others: *Contraceptive technology,* rev ed 16, New York, 1994, Irvington.
Lichtman R, Papera S: *Gynecology—well woman care,* Norwalk, Conn, 1990, Appleton & Lange.

Depo Provera Injection

Description

The most commonly used injectable progestin contraceptive, Depo Provera (or DMPA) has been used for more than 15 years in over 90 countries. It was finally approved for use in the United States in late 1992 and is rapidly becoming popular here as well. Advantages of its use include long-lasting action, requiring only 4-6 injections a year, with minimal impairment of lactation. DMPA shares the advantages that all progestin-only hormonal contraceptives have.

Indications

In breast feeding women there is no adverse effect on lactation, and in fact some studies suggest an increase in milk volume. Depo Provera is generally begun at the 6-week postpartum checkup in lactating women.

In older women Depo Provera is desirable because of the non-estrogen properties, increasing safety. Depo Provera also has low failure rates.

In adolescent or young women Depo Provera is desirable because of its very low failure rate and ready reversibility. The development of thick cervical mucus also imparts some protection against pelvic inflammatory disease.

Depo Provera may be used in women who cannot take estrogen.

Contraindications/Precautions

Depo Provera should not be used if any of the following occur:

- Known or suspected pregnancy
- Unexplained abnormal vaginal bleeding in the past 3 months
- Pregnancy planned in the fairly near future
- Concern over weight gain

Caution should be exercised in prescribing to women with severe, acute liver disease or liver tumors or to women with severe gallbladder disease.

Patient Preparation/Education

Practitioners provide an in-depth discussion of various contraceptive methods and, after DMPA is chosen, detailed patient teaching regarding side effects, advantages, disadvantages, and so on.

Advantages include:

1. No estrogen and therefore no estrogen-related complications such as thrombophlebitis or pulmonary embolism
2. Noncontraceptive benefits, which include:

   - Scanty or no menses
   - Decreases anemia
   - Decreased menstrual cramping and pain
   - Suppression of pain associated with ovulation
   - Decreased risk of endometrial and ovarian cancer
   - Decreased risk of pelvic inflammatory disease
   - Decreased pain associated with endometriosis

3. Reversibility of effects and return to fertility (DMPA has a return time of up to 18 months.)
4. Long-term effective contraception with no day-to-day responsibility

5. Low risk of ectopic pregnancy
6. Amenorrhea

Disadvantages include:

1. Menstrual cycle disturbances: Many women will experience an increase in the number of days they experience light spotting or bleeding. The longer a woman is on DMPA, the greater the probability that she'll experience amenorrhea. Heavy bleeding is uncommon.
2. Weight gain: Some women complain of weight gain or of bloating. World Health Organization statistics depict a 2.2 pound weight gain annually in nearly all women using DMPA. It is felt that most of the weight gain is caused by an increase in appetite rather than fluid retention.
3. Breast tenderness is noted in some women but is not usually severe. Pregnancy always must be ruled out.
4. Bone density loss is seen in both heavy and light women; it seems reversible, but research in this area has been poorly done. More information is needed.

Equipment

- 150 mg DMPA/1 cc
- 21 to 23 gauge, 2.5 to 4 cm needle
- Sterile 3-cc syringe

Procedure

Give the medication deep IM into either the deltoid or the gluteal muscle. Injections into the deltoid may be more socially acceptable, but also may be more painful. DO NOT MASSAGE THE INJECTION SITE, because this may disperse the medication too rapidly and lower DMPA's effectiveness.

Postprocedure patient education

At each 3-month followup visit, ask patients about weight gain and any problems, concerns, or questions the woman may have.

Discuss her risks for STDs and HIV infection; counsel her to use condoms if she is at risk.

Practitioner Followup/Complications

If the patient is late for her injection, the practitioner should try to find out why she has been late. Practitioners help her deal with any barriers she may have encountered (changes in menstrual bleeding pattern, cost, time lost in coming to clinic for injection, partner or family disapproval, etc.). Practitioners stress the importance of returning on time if she chooses to continue DMPA contraception.

Although allergic reactions to DMPA are rare, practitioners should be prepared to deal with anaphylactic reactions by having epinephrine, steroids, and diphenhydramine immediately available.

Menstrual changes are the norm when using DMPA, especially in the first year of use. Practitioners need to be sure to counsel every woman about these effects, because this is the major reason for discontinuation of DMPA contraception. Spotting or breakthrough bleeding can be managed by offering women one or two cycles of combined oral contraceptives. Five days of pills may be enough and may be repeated. It should be reemphasized to the patient that amenorrhea will increase over time and is not harmful; it is in fact viewed as a desired side effect by many women.

CPT BILLING CODE

90782—Therapeutic or diagnostic injection (specify material injected); subcutaneous or intramuscular.

BIBLIOGRAPHY

Cunningham GF, and others: *Williams obstetrics,* ed 19, Norwalk, Conn, 1994, Appleton & Lange.

Hatcher RA, and others: *Contraceptive technology,* rev ed 16, New York, 1994, Irvington.

Checklist for Certification

_____
PROCEDURE

_____
NURSE PRACTITIONER

Procedure process reviewed ———

Reading relevant to procedure completed ———

Procedure observed ———

Completed procedure under direct supervision ———
DATE

    Had equipment ready ———

    Followed correct order of steps ———

    Gave adequate pre-procedure instruction ———

    Gave follow up instruction ———

    Verbalized contraindications ———

    Verbalized how to assess for complications ———

Completed procedure with backup available ———
DATE

Supervision and certification given by qualified expert ———

_____
SIGNATURE CERTIFYING INDIVIDUAL/DATE

Comments: _____

_____

_____

Bibliography

Barker L, Burton J, Zieve P: *Principles of ambulatory medicine,* ed 4, Baltimore, 1995, Williams & Wilkens.

Barkin RM, Rosen P: *Emergency pediatrics, a guide to ambulatory care,* St Louis, 1994, Mosby.

Bates B: *A guide to physical examination,* ed 6, Philadelphia, 1995, Lippincott.

Fischer P and others: *The office laboratory,* East Norwalk, Conn, 1983, Appleton-Century-Crofts.

Fitzpatrick T and others: *Color atlas and synopsis of clinical dermatology,* ed 2, New York, 1992, McGraw-Hill.

Grossman M, Dieckman R: *Pediatric emergency medicine,* Philadelphia, 1991, Lippincott.

Jastremski M: *Emergency procedures,* Philadelphia, 1992, WB Saunders.

Mayhew HE, Rodgers LA: *Basic procedures in family practice, an illustrated manual,* New York, 1984, Wiley Medical.

Perry AG, Potter PA: *Clinical nursing skills and techniques,* ed 3, St Louis, 1994, Mosby.

Pfenninger JL, Fowler GC: *Procedures for primary care physicians,* St Louis, 1994, Mosby.

Proehl JA: *Adult emergency nursing procedures,* Boston, 1993, Jones & Bartlett.

Reisdorff EJ, Roberts MR, Wiegenstein J: *Pediatric emergency medicine,* Philadelphia, 1993, WB Saunders.

Roberts PW: *Useful procedures in medical practice,* Philadelphia, 1987, Lea & Febiger.

Simon RR, Brenner BE: *Emergency procedures and techniques,* ed 3, Baltimore, 1994, Williams & Wilkins.

Index

Page numbers in *ital* include illustrations. Page numbers followed by a t indicate tables.

A

Abdominal aortic aneurysm, 221
Abdominal distention, 172
Abortion, 258
Abscess, 5
    culture and sensitivity testing of material, 48
Abscess incision and drainage
    contraindications/precautions, 49
    description, 48
    equipment, 49–50
    indications, 48
    patient preparation/education, 49
    practitioner followup/complications, 52
        CPT billing codes, 53
    procedure, 50–52, *51*
        postprocedure patient education, 52
Acrochordon, 56
Activated charcoal, medications bound by, *176*
Adjunct therapy, 202–203
Adnexal prolapse, 253
Alkali poisoning, 175
Anal pain, 178
Anemia, 225
Anesthesia
    contraindications/precautions, 21
    description, 20
    equipment
        local, 22
        peripheral nerve block, 22
        topical, 22
    indications, 20–21
    patient preparation/education, 21

Anesthesia—cont'd
    practitioner followup/complications, 27
        CPT billing code, 27
    procedure
        local, 24t, 25–26, *25*
        peripheral nerve block, 26–27, *27*
        postprocedure patient education, 27
        topical, 22, 23t, *25*
    selection of local, *25*
Annular ligament, 218
Anoscopy
    contraindications/precautions, 178
    description, 178
    equipment, 179
    indications, 178
    patient preparation/education, 178
    practitioner followup/complications, 181
        CPT billing codes, 181
    procedure, 179, *179–180*
        postprocedure patient education, 179
Anterior drawer test, *212*
Anterior medial surface, 160
Antireflux valve, 188
Arterial flow, 155
Asthma, 140

B

Bacteremia, 5
Bacteriuria, 17
Barium enema, 182
Barrier contraceptive method, 259
Bartholin glands, 239
Bedside cystometrogram
    contraindications/precautions, 233
    description, 230–231

Bedside cystometrogram—cont'd
equipment, 233–234
indications, 232
patient preparation/education, 233
practitioner followup/complications,
235–236
CPT billing codes, 236
procedure, 234–235
Bethesda system, 240
Biopsy, 184
contraindications/precautions, 43–44
description, 43
equipment, 44
indications, 43
patient preparation/education, 44
practitioner followup/complications,
47–48
CPT billing codes, 48
procedure, 44–45, *44, 45, 46, 47*
postprocedure patient education, 47
Birth control; *see* Cervical cap placement,
Depo Provera injection, Diaphragm fitting
Black dot tinea, 74
Bladder outlet obstruction, 230
Blood cultures
contraindications/precautions, 5–6
description, 5
equipment, 6
indications, 5
patient preparation/education, 6
practitioner followup/complications, 8
CPT billing codes, 8
procedure, 6–8
interpretation of results, 7
postprocedure patient education, 7–8
Borrelia burgdorferi, 79
BUN, 231

C

Calcaneofibular ligament, 209
Callus; *see* Corn management
Candida, 245
Carcinoma, 19
Cardiovascular procedures
Doppler ultrasound of lower extremities,
153–157
contraindications/precautions, 154
description, 153
equipment, 154
indications, 153

Cardiovascular procedures—cont'd
Doppler ultrasound of lower extremities—
cont'd
patient preparation/education, 154
practitioner followup/complications,
157
CPT billing codes, 157
procedure, 154–155, *155, 156*
interpretation of results, 155–156
past procedure patient education,
156–157
electrocardiogram, 158–162
contraindications/precautions, 159
description, 158–159, *158*
equipment, 159–160
indications, 159
patient preparation/education, 159
practitioner followup/complications,
161
CPT billing codes, 161–162
procedure, 160
chest leads, 160, *161*
interpretation of results, 161, *162*
limb leads, 160
postprocedure patient education, 161
Carpal tunnel syndrome, 203
Catheterization, 13
Cellulitis, 5, 75
Certification, checklist for, 273
Cerumen disimpaction
contraindications/precautions, 114–115
description, 113
equipment, 115
indications, 114
patient preparation/education, 115
practitioner followup/complications, 117
CPT billing codes, 117
procedure, 115–117, *116*
postprocedure patient education, *117*
Cervical cap placement
contraindications/precautions, 264–265
description, 263–264, *264*
equipment, 265
indications, 264
patient preparation/education, 265
practitioner followup/complications,
267–268
CPT billing codes, 268
procedure, 265–266
postprocedure patient education,
266–267

Cervix, 238
Chemical destruction of warts, 62–65
Chlamydia, 239, 244
Chronic cystitis, 230
Chronic obstructive pulmonary disease
    (COPD), 137, 140
Coagulopathy, 43
Collateral ligaments, 204
Common warts, 65
Compartment syndrome, 200
Computerized tomography (CT), 222
Condylomata acuminate, treatment of
    contraindications/precautions, 249, 250*t*
    description, 247–248
    equipment, 249
    indications, 248
    patient preparation/education, 249
    practitioner followup/complications, 252
        CPT billing codes, 252–253
    procedure, 249, 251
        postprocedure patient education,
            251–252
Continuous electrocardiography
    contraindications/precautions, 163–164
    description, 163
    equipment, 164
    indications, 163
    patient preparation/education, 164
    practitioner followup/complications, 166
        CPT billing codes, 166
    procedure, 164–165, *165*
        interpretation of results, 165
        postprocedure patient education, 165
Corn and callus management
    contraindications/precautions, 82
    description, 81–82
    equipment, 82–83
    indications, 82
    patient preparation/education, 82
    practitioner followup/complications, 84
        CPT billing codes, 84
    procedure
        postprocedure patient education, 83
        removal of calluses, 83
        removal of hard or soft corns, 83
Corneal abrasions, 99
    treatment of
        contraindications/precautions, 106
        description, 105
            indications, 105–106
        equipment, 107

Corneal abrasions—cont'd
    treatment of—cont'd
        eye conditions that warrant immediate
            referral, *106*
        eye problems that need same-day care,
            106
        patient preparation/education, 107
        practitioner followup/complications,
            110
        procedure, 107–109, *108, 109*
Cornified epithelium, 59
Coronary artery disease, 159
Cortex, 199
Corynebacterium, 7
Creatinine, 231
Crutches, 216
Cryotherapy
    for ankle sprains, 216
    for warts, 65–68
Cultures
    blood, 5–8
    sources of, 1
    urine, 3, 13–18, 14–15*t*
Cyst
    epidermal, 53
    keratinizing, 53
    removal of
        contraindications/precautions, 54
        description, 53
        equipment, 54
        indications, 53
        patient preparation/education, 54
        practitioner followup/complications, 56
            CPT billing codes, 56
        procedure, 55
            postprocedure patient education, 55
    sebaceous, 53
Cystitis, 13
Cystocele, 255*t,* 260
Cystometrogram, bedside, 230–236
Cystometry, 233
Cytobrush, 240

D

Debridement, ulcer, 68–69
Depo Provera injection
    contraindications/precautions, 269
    description, 268
    equipment, 270
    indications, 268–269
    patient preparation/education, 269–270

Depo Provera injection—cont'd
  practitioner followup/complications, 271
    CPT billing codes, 271
  procedure, 270
    postprocedure patient education, 270–271
Dermatologic procedures
  abscess incision and drainage, 48–53
    contraindications/precautions, 49
    description, 48
    equipment, 49–50
    indications, 48
    patient preparation/education, 49
    practitioner followup/complications, 52
      CPT billing codes, 53
    procedure, 50–52, *51*
      postprocedure patient education, 52
  anesthesia, 20–28
    contraindications/precautions, 21
    description, 20
    equipment
      local, 22
      peripheral nerve block, 22
      topical, 22
    indications, 20–21
    local, 24*t,* 25–26, *25*
      peripheral nerve block, 26–27, *27*
      postprocedure patient education, 27
      selection of, *25*
    patient preparation/education, 21
    practitioner followup/complications, 27
      CPT billing code, 27
    procedure, topical, 22, 23*t,* 25
  biopsy, 43–48
    contraindications/precautions, 43–44
    description, 43
    equipment, 44
    indications, 43
    patient preparation/education, 44
    postprocedure patient education, 47
    practitioner followup/complications,
      47–48
      CPT billing codes, 48
    procedure, 44–45, *44, 45, 46,* 47
  corn and callus management, 81–84
    contraindications/precautions, 82
    description, 81–82
    equipment, 82–83
    indications, 82
    patient preparation/education, 82
    practitioner followup/complications, 84
      CPT billing codes, 84

Dermatologic procedures—cont'd
  corn and callus management—cont'd
    procedure, 83
      postprocedure patient education, 83
      removal of calluses, 83
      removal of hard or soft corns, 83
  cyst removal, 53–56
    contraindications/precautions, 54
    description, 53
    equipment, 54
    indications, 53
    patient preparation/education, 54
    practitioner followup/complications, 56
      CPT billing codes, 56
    procedure, 55
      postprocedure patient education, 55
  elliptical excision, 43–48
    contraindications/precautions, 43–44
    description, 43
    equipment, 44
    indications, 43
    patient preparation/education, 44
    postprocedure patient education, 47
    practitioner followup/complications,
      47–48
      CPT billing codes, 48
    procedure, 44–45, *44, 45, 46,* 47
  fungal scraping, 74–78
    contraindications/precautions, 76
    description, 74
    equipment, 76
    indications, 74–75, 75*t*
    patient preparation/education, 76
    practitioner followup/complications, 78
    procedure, 76–77
      interpretation of results, 77–78, *77*
      postprocedure patient education, 78
  ingrown toenail management, 88–94
    contraindications/precautions, 89
    description, 88–89
    equipment
      conservative management, 90
      partial nail removal, 90
    indications, 89
    patient preparation/education, 89
    practitioner followup/complications,
      93–94
      CPT billing codes, 94
    prevention, 93
    procedure
      conservative management, 90–91

Dermatologic procedures—cont'd
  ingrown toenail management—cont'd
    procedure—cont'd
      partial nail removal, 91–92, *92*
      postprocedure patient education,
        92–93
  skin lesion removal, 19–20
  skin tag removal, 56–59
    contraindications/precautions, 57
    description, 56–57
    equipment, 57–58
    indications, 57
    patient preparation/education, 57
    practitioner followup/complications, 59
      CPT billing codes, 59
    procedure, 58
      electrocautery, 58
      postprocedure patient education, 58
      snipping with scissors, 58
  subungual hematoma evacuation, 94–98
    contraindications/precautions, 95
    description, 94–95
    equipment, 95–96
    indications, 95
    patient preparation/education, 95
    practitioner followup/complications, 98
      CPT billing codes, 98
    procedure, 96–97, *97*
      postprocedure patient education,
        97–98
  suturing simple lacerations, 28–43
    care of, *41*
    contraindications/precautions, 29
    description, 28
    equipment, 30, 33–37, *35, 36, 37, 38,
      39, 40*
    indications, 28
    needle selection, *33*
    patient preparation/education, 29, *29*
    postprocedure patient education,
      37–39
    practitioner followup/complications,
      39–42, *41, 42*
      CPT billing codes, 42
    removal, *42*
    selection, *30,* 31–32*t,* 33*t*
  tick removal, 79–81
    contraindications/precautions, 79
    description, 79
    equipment, 79
    indications, 79

Dermatologic procedures—cont'd
  tick removal—cont'd
    practitioner followup/complications,
      80–81
      CPT billing codes, 81
    procedure, 80
  toenail care in diabetic patient, 84–88
    contraindications/precautions, 85
    description, 84
    equipment, 86
    indications, 84–85, *85*
    patient preparation/education, 85–86
    practitioner followup/complications, 88
      CPT billing codes, 88
    procedure, 86, *87*
      postprocedure patient education,
        86–87
  ulcer debridement, 68–71
    contraindications/precautions, 69
    description, 68–69
    equipment, 69
    patient preparation/education, 69
    practitioner followup/complications, 70
      CPT billing codes, 71
    procedure
      postprocedure patient education, 70
      surgical excision, 69–70
      topical agents, 70
  wart removal, 59–68
    chemical destruction
      equipment, 62–63
      patient preparation/education, 62
      practitioner followup/complications,
        65
      procedure, 63–65
    contraindications/precautions, 61–62
    cryotherapy, 65
      equipment, 66
      patient preparation/education, 66
      practitioner followup/complications,
        67–68
      CPT billing codes, 68
      procedure, 66–67
    description, 59–61
    indications, 61
  wound care, 71–74
    contraindications/precautions, 72
    description, 71
    equipment, 72
    indications, 71
    patient preparation/education, 72

Dermatologic procedures—cont'd
  wound care—cont'd
    practitioner followup/complications, 73
    procedure, 73
      postprocedure patient education, 73
Dermatophytes, 74
Dermatophytosis, 77
Detrusor hyperactivity, 231, 234
Detrusor instability, 231
Detrusor weakness, 234
Diabetes, urinalysis during, 9
Diaphragm fitting
  contraindications/precautions, 259–260
  description, 259
  equipment, 260–261
  indications, 259
  patient preparation/education, 260
  practitioner followup/complications, 263
    CPT billing codes, 263
  procedure, 261–262
    postprocedure patient education,
      262–263
Diarrhea, 1
Diethyl stilbestrol (DES), 238
Distal interphalangeal joints, 206
DMPA contraception, 271
Doppler ultrasound of lower extremities
  contraindications/precautions, 154
  description, 153
  equipment, 154
  indications, 153
  patient preparation/education, 154
  practitioner followup/complications, 157
    CPT billing codes, 157
  procedure, 154–155, *155, 156*
    interpretation of results, 155–156
    past procedure patient education,
      156–157
Dressings
  hygroscopic, 70
  occlusive, 70
Dysmenorrhea, 253
Dyspareunia, 253
Dysuria, 13, 14–15*t*
Dysuria syndrome, differential diagnosis of,
  14–15*t*

E

Ear, removal of foreign body from, 110
Ear piercing
  contraindications/precautions, 119

Ear piercing—cont'd
  description, 118
  equipment, 119–120
  indications, 119
  patient preparation/education, 119
  practitioner followup/complications,
    121–122
    CPT billing codes, 122
  procedure, 120–121
    postprocedure patient education, 121
Ecchymoses, 125
Electrocardiogram
  contraindications/precautions, 159
  description, 158–159, *158*
  equipment, 159–160
  indications, 159
  patient preparation/education, 159
  practitioner followup/complications, 161
    CPT billing codes, 161–162
  procedure, 160
    chest leads, 160, *161*
    interpretation of results, 161, *162*
    limb leads, 160
    postprocedure patient education, 161
Electroconductive tags, 160
Elliptical excision
  contraindications/precautions, 43–44
  description, 43
  equipment, 44
  indications, 43
  patient preparation/education, 44
  practitioner followup/complications,
    47–48
    CPT billing codes, 48
  procedure, 44–45, *44, 45, 46,* 47
    postprocedure patient education, 47
Emphysema, 140
Empiric treatment, 3
Endocervical scraping, 240
Endometrium, 237
End-stage dementia, 192
Enteral tube feeding
  contraindications/precautions, 192
  description, 190
  equipment, 193
  indications, 190–192
  patient preparation/education, 192
  practitioner followup/complications, 196
  procedure, 193–194
    feeding instructions, 194–195
    feeding using feeding button, 195

Enteral tube feeding—cont'd
   procedure—cont'd
      postprocedure patient education,
         195–196
Epidermal cyst, 53
Epistaxis and nasal packing
   contraindications/precautions, 123–124
   description, 122–123, *123*
   equipment, 125–126
   indications, 123
   patient preparation/education, 124–125,
      125
   practitioner followup/complications, 129
   procedure, 126–127, *128*
      postprocedure patient education, 127,
         129
Erythema migrans, 80
Erythrasma, 78
Estrogen deprivation, 230
Eversion injuries, 210
Eye, ear, and nose procedures
   cerumen disimpaction, 113–118
      contraindications/precautions, 114–115
      description, 113
      equipment, 115
      indications, 114
      patient preparation/education, 115
      practitioner followup/complications,
         117
         CPT billing codes, 117
      procedure, 115–117, *116*
         postprocedure patient education, 117
   corneal abrasion, treatment of
      contraindications/precautions, 106
      description, 105
      indications, 105–106
      equipment, 107
      eye conditions that warrant immediate
         referral, *106*
      eye problems that need same-day care,
         106
      patient preparation/education, 107
      practitioner followup/complications,
         110
      procedure, 107–109, *108, 109*
   ear piercing, 118–122
      contraindications/precautions, 119
      description, 118
      equipment, 119–120
      indications, 119
      patient preparation/education, 119

Eye, ear, and nose procedures—cont'd
   ear piercing—cont'd
      practitioner followup/complications,
         121–122
      CPT billing codes, 122
      procedure, 120–121
         postprocedure patient education, 121
   epistaxis and nasal packing, 122–130
      contraindications/precautions, 123–124
      description, 122–123, *123*
      equipment, 125–126
      indications, 123
      patient preparation/education, 124–125,
         125
      practitioner followup/complications,
         129
      procedure, 126–127, *128*
         postprocedure patient education, 127,
            129
   foreign body
      removal of, from ear
         contraindications/precautions, 111
         description, 110
         equipment, 111
         indications, 110
         patient preparation/education, 111
         practitioner followup/complications,
            113
         CPT billing codes, 113
         procedure, 111–112, *112*
            postprocedure patient education,
               112–113
      removal of, from eye
         contraindications/precautions, 100
         description, 99
         equipment, 101
         indications, 99–100
         patient preparation/education,
            100–101
         practitioner followup/complications,
            105
         procedure
            examination, 101–103, *102, 104*
            postprocedure patient education,
               103–105
            preparation, 101
      removal of, from nose
         contraindications/precautions, 131
         description, 130
         equipment, 132, *132*
         indications, 131

Eye, ear, and nose procedures—cont'd
  foreign body—cont'd
    removal of, from nose—cont'd
      patient preparation/education, 131
      practitioner followup/complications,
        135–136
      procedure, 133–134, *134, 135*
        postprocedure patient education,
          134–135
Eye, removal of foreign body from
  contraindications/precautions, 100
  description, 99
  equipment, 101
  indications, 99–100
  patient preparation/education, 100–101
  procedure
    examination, 101–103, *102, 104*
    postprocedure patient education,
      103–105
    preparation, 101

F

Fecal incontinence, 182
Filiform warts, 60
Finger stick blood glucose
  contraindications/precautions, 225
  description, 224
  equipment, 225–226
  indications, 224–225
  patient preparation/education, 225
  practitioner followup/complications, 229
  procedure, 226–228
    interpretation of results, 228–229
    postprocedure patient education, 228
Focused light source, 239
Foreign body
  removal of, from ear
    contraindications/precautions, 111
    description, 110
    equipment, 111
    indications, 110
    patient preparation/education, 111
    practitioner followup/complications,
      113
    CPT billing codes, 113
    procedure, 111–112, *112*
      postprocedure patient education,
        112–113
  removal of, from eye
    contraindications/precautions, 100
    description, 99

Foreign body—cont'd
  removal of, from eye—cont'd
    equipment, 101
    indications, 99–100
    patient preparation/education, 100–101
    practitioner followup/complications,
      105
    procedure
      examination, 101–103, *102, 104*
      postprocedure patient education,
        103–105
      preparation, 101
  removal of, from nose
    contraindications/precautions, 131
    description, 130
    equipment, 132, *132*
    indications, 131
    patient preparation/education, 131
    practitioner followup/complications,
      135–136
    procedure, 133–134, *134, 135*
      postprocedure patient education,
        134–135
Fowler's position, 168
Fracture immobilization
  contraindications/precautions, 200
  description, 199
  equipment, 201
  indications, 200
  patient preparation/education, 200–201
  practitioner followup/complications, 202
    CPT billing codes, 202
  procedure, 201
    postprocedure patient education, 202
Fungal scraping
  contraindication/precautions, 76
  description, 74
  equipment, 76
  indications, 74–75, *75t*
  patient preparation/education, 76
  practitioner followup/complications, 78
  procedure, 76–77
    interpretation of results, 77–78, *77*
    postprocedure patient education, 78
Fungemia, 5

G

Gastric lavage
  contraindications/precautions, 175
  description, 174
  equipment, 175–176

Gastric lavage—cont'd
  indications, 174
  patient preparation/education, 175
  practitioner followup/complications, 177
    CPT billing codes, 177–178
  procedure, 176–177
Gastrocolic reflex, 184
Gastrointestinal procedures
  anoscopy, 178–181
    contraindications/precautions, 178
    description, 178
    equipment, 179
    indications, 178
    patient preparation/education, 178
    practitioner followup/complications,
      181
      CPT billing codes, 181
    procedure, 179, *179–180*
      postprocedure patient education,
        179
  enteral tube feeding, 190–198
    contraindications/precautions, 192
    description, 190
    equipment, 193
    indications, 190–192
    patient preparation/education, 192
    procedure, 193–194
      feeding instructions, 194–195
      feeding using feeding button, 195
      postprocedure patient education,
        195–196
  gastric lavage, 174–178
    contraindications/precautions, 175
    description, 174
    equipment, 175–176
    indications, 174
    patient preparation/education, 175
    practitioner followup/complications,
      177
      CPT billing codes, 177–178
    procedure, 176–177
  nasogastric tube insertion and removal,
    167–174
    contraindications/precautions, 167–168
    description, 167
    equipment, 168–169
    indications, 167
    patient preparation/education, 168
    practitioner followup/complications,
      173
      CPT billing codes, 173–174

Gastrointestinal procedures—cont'd
  nasogastric tube insertion and removal—
    cont'd
    procedure, 169–170, *171, 172*
      criteria for removal of nasogastric
        tube, 172–173
      removal of nasogastric tube, 173
  percutaneous endoscopic gastrostomy tube
    (PEG) management, 185–190
    contraindications/precautions, 186
    description, 185, *185, 186*
    equipment, 187
    indications, 186
    patient preparation/education, 186–187
    practitioner followup/complications,
      187–190
    procedure, postprocedure patient educa-
      tion, 187
  rectal prolapse reduction, 181–185
    description, 181–182
    equipment, 182
    indications, 182
    practitioner followup/complications,
      184
    procedure, 183
      postprocedure patient education,
        183–184
Gonorrhea, 239, 244
Gram's stain results, 3
Gynecologic procedures
  cervical cap placement, 263–268
    contraindications/precautions, 264–265
    description, 263–264, *264*
    equipment, 265
    indications, 264
    patient preparation/education, 265
    practitioner followup/complications,
      267–268
      CPT billing codes, 268
    procedure, 265–266
      postprocedure patient education,
        266–267
  Condylomata acuminate, treatment of
    contraindications/precautions, 249, 250*t*
    description, 247–248
    equipment, 249
    indications, 248
    patient preparation/education, 249
    practitioner followup/complications,
      252
      CPT billing codes, 252–253

Gynecologic procedures—cont'd
  Condylomata acuminate, treatment of—
      cont'd
    procedure, 249, 251
      postprocedure patient education,
          251–252
  Depo Provera injection, 268–271
    contraindications/precautions, 269
    description, 268
    equipment, 270
    indications, 268–269
    patient preparation/education, 269–270
    practitioner followup/complications,
        271
      CPT billing codes, 271
    procedure, 270
      postprocedure patient education,
          270–271
  diaphragm fitting, 259–263
    contraindications/precautions, 259–
        260
    description, 259
    equipment, 260–261
    indications, 259
    patient preparation/education, 260
    practitioner followup/complications,
        263
      CPT billing codes, 263
    procedure, 261–262
      postprocedure patient education,
          262–263
  Papanicolaou smear test, 237–242
    contraindications/precautions, 238
    description, 237
    equipment, 239
    indications, 237–238
    patient preparation/education, 238
    practitioner followup/complications,
        242
      CPT billing codes, 242
    procedure, 239–240
      indications for colposcopy, 241
      interpretation of results, 240–241
      postprocedure patient education,
          241–242
  pessary use, 253–259
    contraindications/precautions, 254
    description, 253
    equipment, 255t, 256
    indications, 253–254
      obstetrical, 254

Gynecologic procedures—cont'd
  pessary use—cont'd
    patient preparation/education, 254
    practitioner followup/complications,
        258
      CPT billing codes, 258–259
    procedure, 256–258, 256, 257
      postprocedure patient education, 258
  treatment of condylomata acuminata,
      247–253
  wet mount, 242–247
    contraindications/precautions, 243
    description, 242–243
    equipment, 243–244
    indications, 243
    patient preparation/education, 243
    practitioner followup/complications,
        247
      CPT billing codes, 247
    procedure, 244–245
      interpretation of results, 245, 246t
      postprocedure patient education, 247

H

Hematoma, subungual, evacuation of, 94 –98
Hemorrhoids, 178
Hernia, 253
Herpes, 239
Hiccups, 110
Holter monitoring; *see* Continuous electro-
    cardiography
Hygroscopic dressings, 70
Hyperglycemia, 224
Hypoglycemia, 224
Hypotension, orthostatic, 125

I

Ingrown toenail management
    contraindications/precautions, 89
    description, 88–89
    equipment, 90
    indications, 89
    patient preparation/education, 89
    practitioner followup/complications,
        93–94
      CPT billing codes, 94
    prevention, 93
    procedure, 90–91
      conservative management, 90–91
      partial nail removal, 90, 91–92, 92
      postprocedure patient education, 92–93

Inoculum, 7
Intraabdominal air fluid levels, 221
Intraabdominal pressure, 230
Ipecac syrup, 174

J

Jejunostomy, 192

K

Keratinizing cyst, 53
Kerions, 75
Kisselbach's plexus, 122
KOH test, 78; *see also* Fungal scraping

L

Lacerations, suturing simple, 28–42
Latex allergy, 259
Leukocyte esterase, 3
Ligament injury, clinical diagnosis of, 211*t*
Liquid nitrogen, 65
Lithotomy position, 243
Little's area, 122
Lyme disease, 79, 80

M

Malnutrition, 190
Medial malleolar sprains, 210
Medullary canal, 199
Melanocytic nevus, 57
Menorrhagia, 253
Metabolic/miscellaneous procedures
  bedside cystometrogram, 230–236
    contraindications/precautions, 233
    description, 230–231
    equipment, 233–234
    indications, 232
    patient preparation/education, 233
    practitioner followup/complications,
      235–236
    CPT billing codes, 236
    procedure, 234–235
  finger stick blood glucose, 224–230
    contraindications/precautions, 225
    description, 224
    equipment, 225–226
    indications, 224–225
    patient preparation/education, 225
    practitioner followup/complications,
      229
    procedure, 226–228
      interpretation of results, 228–229

Metabolic/miscellaneous procedures—cont'd
  finger stick blood glucose—cont'd
    procedure—cont'd
      postprocedure patient education, 228
  x-ray interpretation, 221–224
    contraindications/precautions, 221–222
    description, 221
    indications, 221
    procedure
      bony films, 223
      chest x-ray exam, 222
      interpretation of results, 223
      postprocedure patient education,
        223–224
Metacarpophalangeal joint, 204
Metoclopramide, 192
Miscarriage, 258
Molluscum contagiosum, 57
Musculoskeletal procedures
  bedside cystometrogram
    contraindications/precautions, 233
    description, 230–231
    equipment, 233–234
    indications, 232
    patient preparation/education, 233
    practitioner followup/complications,
      235–236
    CPT billing codes, 236
    procedure, 234–235
  fracture immobilization, 199–202
    contraindications/precautions, 200
    description, 199
    equipment, 201
    indications, 200
    patient preparation/education, 200–201
    practitioner followup/complications,
      202
    CPT billing codes, 202
    procedure, 201
      postprocedure patient education, 202
  reduction of subluxed radial head,
    218–220
  splinting–ankle sprains, 209–217
    contraindications/precautions, 212–213,
      212
    description, 209–210, *209, 210*
    equipment, 214
    indications, 210, 211*t*
    patient preparation/education, 213–214
    practitioner followup/complications, 217
    CPT billing codes, 217

Musculoskeletal procedures—cont'd
  splinting–ankle sprains—cont'd
    procedure, 214–217
    specific tests, *212*
  splinting–hand and wrist
    contraindications/precautions, 203
    description, 202–203
    equipment, 203–204
    indications, 203
    patient preparation/education, 203
    practitioner followup/complications, 208
      CPT billing codes, 208
    procedure, 204, *205*, 206–207, *206, 207*
      postprocedure patient education, 207
  subluxed radial head, reduction of
    contraindications/precautions, 218
    description, 218
    indications, 218
    patient preparation/education, 218
    practitioner followup/complications, 219
      CPT billing codes, 219
    procedure, 219
      postprocedure patient education, 219
Mycobacteria, 1
Myocardial infarction, 161

N

Nasogastric feeding, 191
Nasogastric tube (NGT), 167
  insertion and removal
    contraindications/precautions, 167–168
    description, 167
    equipment, 168–169
    indications, 167
    patient preparation/education, 168
    practitioner followup/complications, 173
      CPT billing codes, 173–174
    procedure, 169–173, *171, 172*
      criteria for removal of nasogastric tube, 172–173
      removal of nasogastric tube, 173
Nasopulmonary reflexes, 124
Nebulizer treatment
  contraindications/precautions, 137–138
  description, 137
  equipment, 138
  indications, 137

Nebulizer treatment—cont'd
  patient preparation/education, 138
  postprocedure patient education, 139
  practitioner followup/complications, 139
  procedure, 138
Neurovascular compromise, 201, 207
Nocturia, 13
Nonsteroidal antiinflammatory medications (NSAIDs), 216
Nosebleeds, 122, 123

O

Occlusive dressing, 70
Ocular injury, 99
Onychocryptosis, 88, 89
Onychogryposis, 89
Onycholysis, 98
Onychomycosis, 89
Oral airway insertion
  contraindications/precautions, 147
  description, 146
  equipment, 148
  indications, 146–147
  patient preparation/education, 147
  practitioner followup/complications, 150–151
  procedure, 148–149, *149*
    nasopharyngeal airway, 150, *150*
    postprocedure patient education, 150
Organomegaly, 125
Oropharyngeal airway, 146
Oropharynx, 170
Orthostatic hypotension, 125
Osteochrondritis dessicans of the talus, 212
Osteomyelitis, 212
Osteopenia, 199
Osteoporosis, 199
Otoscope, 115

P

Papanicolaou smear test
  contraindications/precautions, 238
  description, 237
  equipment, 239
  indications, 237–238
  patient preparation/education, 238
  practitioner followup/complications, 242
    CPT billing codes, 242
  procedure, 239–240
    indications for colposcopy, 241

Papanicolaou smear test—cont'd
  procedure—cont'd
    interpretation of results, 240–241
    postprocedure patient education,
      241–242
Papilloma, pedunculated, 56
Paronychia, 88, 89
Pedunculated papilloma, 56
Pelvic inflammatory disease, 269
Percutaneous endoscopic gastrostomy tube
    (PEG) management
  contraindications/precautions, 186
  description, 185, 185, 186
  equipment, 187
  indications, 186
  patient preparation/education, 186–187
  practitioner followup/complications,
    187–190
  procedure, postprocedure patient educa-
    tion, 187
Perianal pain, 178
Periungual warts, 59–60, 61
Pessary use
  contraindications/precautions, 254
  description, 253
  equipment, 255t, 256
  indications, 253–254
    obstetrical, 254
  patient preparation/education, 254
  practitioner followup/complications, 258
    CPT billing codes, 258–259
  procedure, 256–258, 256, 257
    postprocedure patient education, 258
Petechiae, 125
Photophobia, 106
Physical therapy for ankle sprain, 216
Plantar warts, 59–60, 61, 65
Pneumonia, 1
Podofilox solution, 251
Polarity, 158–159
Polycythemia, 225, 229
Posterior fornix, 261
Postvoid residual, 232
Pregnancy, urinalysis during, 9
Proctoscopy, 182
Progestrin-only hormonal contraceptives,
    268
Proteinuria, urinalysis during, 9
Proximal fifth metatarsal, 212
Proximal interphalangeal, 204

Pseudomonas, 100
Pulmonary disease, 221
Pyelonephritis, 17

R
Raynaud's disease, 225
Rectal prolapse
  reduction of
    description, 181–182
    equipment, 182
    indications, 182
    practitioner followup/complications,
      184–185
    procedure, 183
      postprocedure patient education,
        183–184
  types of, 181
Rectocele, 255t, 260
Respiratory procedures
  nebulizer treatment, 137–139
    contraindications/precautions, 137–138
    description, 137
    equipment, 138
    indications, 137
    patient preparation/education, 138
    postprocedure patient education, 139
    practitioner followup/complications,
      139
    procedure, 138
  oral airway insertion, 146–151
    contraindications/precautions, 147
    description, 146
    equipment, 148
    indications, 146–147
    patient preparation/education, 147
    practitioner followup/complications,
      150–151
    procedure, 148–149, 149
      nasopharyngeal airway, 150, 150
      postprocedure patient education, 150
  spirometry, 139–146
    contraindications/precautions, 140
    description, 139–140
    indications, 140
    patient preparation/education, 140–141
    practitioner followup/complications,
      143–144
      CPT billing codes, 144, 146
    procedure, 141–142
      interpretation of results, 142

Respiratory procedures—cont'd
  spirometry—cont'd
    procedure—cont'd
      interpretation of spirometry made
        easy, 142–143, *143–145*
      postprocedure patient education, 143
Rhinitis
  allergic, 123
  bacterial, 123
  viral, 123
RICE regimen, 214
Rickettsia rickettsii, 79
Rocky Mountain spotted fever, 79, 80

S

Scaling, 74
Sebaceous cyst, 53
Seborrheic keratosis, 57
Septicemia, 5
Septic joint, 212
Sexually transmitted disease (STD), 259
Sigmoidoscopy, 184
Sinus ostia, 136
Skeins gland, 239
Skin lesion removal, 19–20, *20*
Skin tags, 19
  removal of
    contraindications/precautions, 57
    description, 56–57
    equipment, 57–58
    indications, 57
    patient preparation/education, 57
    practitioner followup/complications, 59
      CPT billing codes, 59
    procedure
      electrocautery, 58
      postprocedure patient education, 58
      snipping with scissors, 58
Snoring, 147
Sore throat, 1
Specimen collection
  contraindications/precautions, 2
  description, 1
  equipment, 3
  indications, 2
  patient preparation/education, 2–3
  practitioner followup/complications, 4
  procedure, 3–4
Spirometry
  contraindications/precautions, 140
  description, 139–140

Spirometry—cont'd
  indications, 140
  patient preparation/education, 140–141
  practitioner followup/complications,
    143–144
    CPT billing codes, 144, 146
  procedure, 141–142
    interpretation of results, 142
    interpretation of spirometry made easy,
      142–143, *143–145*
    postprocedure patient education, 143
Splinting
  ankle sprains
    contraindications/precautions, 212–213,
      212
    description, 209–210, *209, 210*
    equipment, 214
    indications, 210, 211*t*
    patient preparation/education, 213–214
    practitioner followup/complications,
      217
      CPT billing codes, 217
    procedure, 214–217
    specific tests, *212*
  hand and wrist
    contraindications/precautions, 203
    description, 202–203
    equipment, 203–204
    indications, 203
    patient preparation/education, 203
    practitioner followup/complications,
      208
      CPT billing codes, 208
    procedure, 204, *205,* 206–207, *206, 207*
      postprocedure patient education, 207
Staphylococcus epidermidis, 3, 7
Stomahesive powder, 188
Subluxed radial head, reduction of
  contraindications/precautions, 218
  description, 218
  indications, 218
  patient preparation/education, 218
  practitioner followup/complications, 219
    CPT billing codes, 219
  procedure, 219
    postprocedure patient education, 219
Subungual hematoma evacuation
  contraindications/precautions, 95
  description, 94–95
  equipment, 95–96
  indications, 95

Subungual hematoma evacuation—cont'd
  patient preparation/education, 95
  practitioner followup/complications, 98
    CPT billing codes, 98
  procedure, 96–97, 97
    postprocedure patient education, 97–98
Surgical excision, 68
Suturing simple lacerations
  care of, 41
  contraindications/precautions, 29
  description, 28
  equipment, 30, 33–37, 35, 36, 37, 38, 39,
    40
  indications, 28
  needle selection, 33
    postprocedure patient education,
      37–39
  patient preparation/education, 29, 29
  practitioner followup/complications,
    39–42, 41, 42
    complications, 40–41
    CPT billing codes, 42
  removing, 42
  suture selection, 30, 31–32t, 33t

T

Talar tilt test, 212
Talofibular ligament, 209
Telangiectasia, 125
Tendinitis, 203
Tenosynovitis, 203
Thompson test, 212
Tick removal
  contraindications/precautions, 79
  description, 79
  equipment, 79
  indications, 79
  practitioner followup/complications,
    80–81
    CPT billing code, 81
  procedure, 80
Tinea capitis, 77
Tinea versicolor, 77
Tinnitus, 117
Toenail
  care of, in diabetic patient
    contraindications/precautions, 85
    description, 84
    equipment, 86
    indications, 84–85, 85
    patient preparation/education, 85–86

Toenail—cont'd
  care of, in diabetic patient—cont'd
    practitioner followup/complications, 88
      CPT billing codes, 88
    procedure, 86, 87
      postprocedure, 86–87
  management of ingrown, 88–94
    contraindications/precautions, 89
    description, 88–89
    equipment
      conservative management, 90
      partial nail removal, 90
    indications, 89
    patient preparation/education, 89
    practitioner followup/complications,
      93–94
      CPT billing codes, 94
    prevention, 93
    procedure
      conservative management, 90–91
      partial nail removal, 91–92, 92
      postprocedure patient education,
        92–93
Topical debriding agents, 68–69
Toxic shock syndrome, 260, 265, 267
Trauma, as cause of nosebleeds in children,
  122
Trichomonas, 245

U

Ulcer debridement
  contraindications/precautions, 69
  description, 68–69
  equipment, 69
  patient preparation/education, 69
  practitioner followup/complications, 70
    CPT billing codes, 71
  procedure
    postprocedure patient education, 70
    surgical excision, 69–70
    topical debriding agents, 70
Ultrasound; see Doppler ultrasound of lower
  extremities
Urinalysis, 231
  contraindications/precautions, 9
  description, 8
  equipment, 9–10
  indications, 9
  patient preparation/education, 9
  practitioner followup/complications, 12
    CPT billing codes, 12

Urinalysis—cont'd
  procedure, 10–12
    chemical examination, 11
    microscopic examination, 11–12
    physical examination, 11
    postprocedure patient education, 12
Urinary incontinence, 230
Urinary tract infections (UTI), 13, 235
Urine cultures, 3, 231
  contraindications/precautions, 13
  description, 13
  equipment, 16
  indications, 13
  patient preparation/education, 13, 16
  practitioner followup/complications, 17
    CPT billing codes, 17
  procedure, 16–17
    interpretation of results, 17
    postprocedure patient education, 17
Uterine prolapse, 253, 265
Uterine retroposition, 253

V

Vaginal, 258
Vaginal abrasions, 258, 267
Vaginal lacerations, 258, 267
Vaginitis, 245
Vascular plexus, 122
Vasoconstriction, 130
Veneral warts; *see* Condylomata acuminata, treatment of
Venous flow, 155
Verrucae; *see* Wart removal
Vulva, 237

W

Warts
  filiform, 60
  periungual, 59–60
  plantar, 59–60
  removal
    chemical destruction
      equipment, 62–63
      patient preparation/education, 62
      practitioner followup/complications, 65
      procedure, 63–65
      contraindications/precautions, 61–62

Warts—cont'd
  removal—cont'd
    cryotherapy, 65
      equipment, 66
      patient preparation/education, 66
      practitioner followup/complication 67–68
        CPT billing codes, 68
      procedure, 66–67
    description, 59, 61
    indications, 61
  types of treatment available for, *60*
Wet mount
  contraindications/precautions, 243
  description, 242–243
  equipment, 243–244
  indications, 243
  patient preparation/education, 243
  practitioner followup/complications, 247
    CPT billing codes, 247
  procedure, 244–245
    interpretation of results, 245, 246*t*
    postprocedure patient education, 247
Wood's lamp test, 74, 77
World Health Organization (WHO), 270
Wound care
  contraindications/precautions, 72
  description, 71
  equipment, 72
  indications, 71
  patient preparation/education, 72
  practitioner followup/complications, 7
  procedure, postprocedure patient educa tion, 73

X

X-ray interpretation
  contraindications/precautions, 221–22
  description, 221
  indications, 221
  procedure
    bony films, 223
    chest x-ray exam, 222
    interpretation of results, 223
    postprocedure patient education, 223–224
X-ray radiogram, 130